THE BABY REFLUX LADY'S SURVIVAL GUIDE

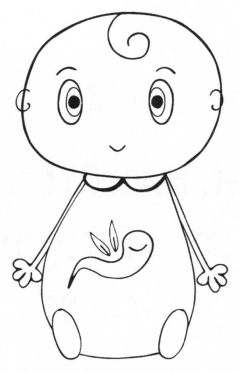

the baby reflux lady

Follow me on Instagram for even more daily learning & please share and tag me with your progress

⊙ @babyrefluxlady

THE BABY REFLUX LADY'S SURVIVAL GUIDE

HOW TO UNDERSTAND & SUPPORT YOUR UNSETTLED BABY AND YOURSELF

Áine Homer

For parents of infants with colic, reflux, silent reflux, CMPA, and other food intolerances and allergies.

Editing by Kris Emery Editorial – www.KrisEmery.com

Illustrations by Ninocka Design

Cover by Imran Shaikh (Retina99)

eBook ISBN: 9781999957445

Paperback ISBN: 9781999957452

First Edition: February 2018
Second Edition: August 2018

For J, Sunflower & Daffodil

TABLE OF CONTENTS

PREFACE

I remember leaving the hospital with my first-born. She was so small I had to pad out the infant car seat to keep her upright. It was snowing and I watched every step my husband J took as he carried her through the crowded hospital. We have never been so cautious crossing a road in our lives, and the 20-minute drive home took almost an hour with the uber-careful driving of a new dad. When we got home, we took her out of the car seat. We looked; nay gazed at her. And that's when he whispered to me, "Where's the instruction manual?" He wasn't joking. He was petrified.

Here we were, two socialites who knew how to party, enjoy life, and trust our in-built homing beacon to get us back from the bar at 3am. Here we were responsible for another human being. Another life. Totally responsible. And that was scary. Life had changed. We'd known it would, but we'd had no idea by how much.

Just 12 hours earlier, I'd had my first night as a mum in a hospital with my baby. My labour had been a night event, so I'd had zero hours' sleep on the Friday night. Baby Sunflower was born at 7:30am, and I was so high on every kind of emotion that I didn't sleep at all during the day. Hubby was kicked out of the hospital at 7pm and I was left to fend for the two of us. Alone. Sunflower, in the bedside cot, wasn't best pleased lying on her own. Frankly, I didn't blame her. I picked her up, listening to my instincts, despite midwives coming in and out telling me to put her down and get some rest. I couldn't leave her. Eventually, exhaustion set in, and I just had to put her down. She had a feed and fell asleep. When I popped her into the cot, she woke immediately. I picked her up again, she settled immediately. I put her down again... The cycle repeated itself for half an hour until she didn't settle when I picked her up. She wanted more milk, so again I fed her.

We played the game over and over for 3 hours...

As early as that first night, I doubted myself. Crying from exhaustion, I couldn't understand why my baby wouldn't sleep. I got up and walked the corridors with her, worried she was starving, worried she was tired, worried because I couldn't help her sleep. I sang to her. I cried with her.

I asked for help and all I got was: "Your baby is disturbing the rest of the ward. Can you go somewhere else please?" She was only 16 hours old.

After my third walk around, she settled on my shoulder, and I climbed back onto my bed holding her. She slept with me, in my arms, waking every 30 minutes for more milk.

By the time J came into us the next morning, I looked awful, felt awful, and after the worst night of my life with zero support, just wanted to go home.

Why do I tell you this story? Well, this was the start of a journey that would transform how I thought about food, its impact on me and my baby, and how I would feed and nourish my child (now children) to give them the best start in life. All that was ahead of me. We would go on to have months of sleepless nights, without any helpful information from GPs, midwifes, lactation consultants, health visitors, or anyone else we thought should know. I was told time and time again: "You're going to have to let her cry and learn to sleep". And my friends didn't understand either. How could they? They had babies who would sleep for 3 to 5 hours at a time, most of whom were sleeping 8 hours straight by 12 weeks! Sure, they were as supportive as they could be, but it's still hard when you feel your life is shit and all your friends are having a breeze. I worried constantly about what my sister thought of me. She had a daughter a year older than Sunflower who would sleep wherever and whenever. My daughter wouldn't even sleep in the car seat, buggy or cot, only on my shoulder, or with her dad on the odd extremely exhausted occasion. But he couldn't be up all night. He had to function, go to work so that we could pay the mortgage and eat.

At this point, I didn't know it would take over 5 months of living like this to figure out what was going on for us. That revelation was a chance happening on a webpage, during one of my regular internet frenzies. (Google was my closest ally.) I found a list of symptoms on a website that described my daughter Sunflower to a T. Finally, I'd found it. She had silent reflux. 100%. I was certain. I rang my GP the next morning to talk through what I should do, or even check if my diagnosis was close. During the conversation, my GP said it sounded "likely that it could be silent reflux" in a condescending manner that a struggling mum really didn't need.

A month later, I found out that I had a leaky gut, which prompted loads more reading, loads more thinking. I changed my diet, gradually at first, which gave some positive results, though not enough to change my life. Consequently, I went on a massive elimination diet, kept a detailed food and symptom diary, and over the course of the next few weeks started to see real change.

At first, my baby's painful gas and bloating reduced; it was no longer taking 2 to 3 hours for her to pass wind. Then, waking periods shortened so we both got more sleep. Later, the gas stopped completely, but baby still fed through the night eight or nine times! (I had an app and was addicted to recording everything, so I know this is no exaggeration.) Those feeds were shorter, though, just 5 minutes each. I'd also mastered the art of side-lying breastfeeding. Sunflower was beside me, so I didn't have to go far to feed her. And most importantly for my sanity, my feet didn't touch the floor during the night.

If you see your own experience in this story, if you have sleepless nights, if you've been given useless information, if you don't know where to turn for help, if you know your baby isn't "manipulating you" to pick them up, you are in the right place. If your professional support has not been the support you hoped it would be, this book could be the answer to taking control of your life and figuring out what's going on for you both.

Remember: babies *do not* manipulate. They use crying to *communicate*. They need closeness. They need support. If they are uncomfortable in any way, they need their mum or dad. You *do not* have to ever deny this contact to your child.

The discomfort is *real*. The symptoms are real. If your baby has any of the following, it could be a sign of a food issue:

- doesn't sleep well or at all
- ongoing frequent feeding (30 to 90 minutes between feeds)
- reflux
- frequent spitting up
- poor weight gain, weight loss or excessive weight gain
- colic
- dry skin, eczema, psoriasis, hives, sore bum, itchy rashes
- constant runny nose, congestion, cold-like symptoms
- breathing difficulties, asthma
- ear infections, glue ear
- fussiness, irritability
- bloating, gas, trapped wind, constipation, diarrhoea, green stools, blood or mucus in stools
- red itchy eyes.

If baby is suffering from any of the above, I suggest you don't hesitate in making an appointment with a paediatric allergist to have your baby checked for intolerance to a wide range of food stuffs. It is vital to understand if baby is intolerant or even allergic to foods. And these two are very different. An allergy initiates a response from the immune system when it encounters something normally considered harmless. The response tends to be immediate (minutes to 2 hours) and severe regardless of the amount of the substance encountered. By contrast, an intolerance does not usually involve the immune system, but rather causes an unpleasant reaction, such as bloating, gas, rashes. Effects are rarely immediate, which make it more challenging to identify the specific culprit or culprits.

Regardless of what your baby's reaction is, if you ***ever*** feel overly concerned or worried, contact your GP or emergency services, or take baby to A&E. In my experience (and I've had a few trips), you will not be turned away or told you're overreacting by any professional when dealing with children and health issues. It is ***always*** better to be safe than sorry.

To read about some of my unnecessary trips to hospital (during none of which I was told I shouldn't have gone in), go to www.ainehomer.com. I have had the full support of medical professionals and I will always err on the side of caution. I share these stories to make you more comfortable with taking similar steps.

If you need help *now*, go to page 5 and read through the table *Where Do I Start?*

This will kick-start a change in your life experience in the next few days. Get more sleep. Look after yourself and your baby first. And trust your instincts. *You* are the expert on *your* child, regardless of anyone else's qualifications.

Now, of course, I don't expect everybody who reads this book to buy all organic food, consume only organic grass-fed free-range meat, become vegetarian or vegan or not. I don't expect you to completely avoid sugar or give up gluten and wheat. What this book is setting out to achieve is providing parents with the right information so you can make the best decisions for your life and family.

Informed decisions are much better than sweeping generalisations made by governments and just accepted by the public to be true, right, and in the best interests of everybody's health. Unfortunately, governments do not always have the right information to hand. Sometimes the information they do have provides a solution that is too expensive to push out to the public, or could cost the economy money, which in turn means lobbying from the food industry. If you think the food industry does not have a large part to play in the health of you and your child, you may need another education.

The guidelines throughout this book are general in nature too. It is *your* decision what you feed your child. However, without this information, all your decisions are made in the dark. If you want to remain in the dark about how food impacts the body of your child and your own body, stop reading right here! On the other hand, if you want to do the very best for your child and their development in every way shape and form, please read on.

WHERE DO I START?

Quickly find the most relevant section for you to jump into *right now* according to your current circumstances. Find the description that fits your situation best and head straight to the appropriate page.

Your Situation	Where to Start
If life is overwhelming, if you feel nothing is right, no-one understands and no-one listens or supports you	Go to the back of the book. Read the section on relationships.
If you feel alone	Know you are not alone. Start at the back and read the stories from other mums.
If you have a new baby (under 2 weeks) who is or has been unsettled since birth; who never really settles for more than an hour or two, sometimes only 30 minutes; who is genuinely up all night, every night, without fail, and cries a lot	Read the whole of Section 1 First Steps (page 8) and then 2.1 What If Baby Just Won't Settle? (page 21).
If you have a baby under 2 weeks with constant large amounts of projectile vomit and still losing weight	Read Section 4.10.13 Pyloric Stenosis (page 106) and phone your GP.
If you have a baby over 2 weeks with constant unsettled behaviour; perhaps has already been diagnosed as "colicky", "needs to learn how to sleep", "fussy", "reflux" or you have had reason enough to pick up this book	Read Section 3.2 Red Flag Symptoms (page 36) first and reassure yourself that there is nothing too serious ongoing. If you are concerned, contact your GP. Once happy that your baby does not have any of these symptoms, read Section 4.2 Cause Or Effect? (page 54) and try to figure out the source of your baby's troubles. This is how you will then start to understand the appropriate solution for your baby.
If you have a baby diagnosed with reflux, maybe taking medication	Most important now is to figure out what is causing your baby's reflux. This is my suggested order:

and you've tried several changes of milk with no real improvement or baby is still experiencing some reflux symptoms	Read Section 4.2 Cause Or Effect? (page 54) to help figure out the cause of your baby's reflux Read Section 5 Anatomy That Impacts Life (page 109) to understand your baby's natural digestive maturity Read Section 6 What's In Baby's Milk? (page 125) to see if any of it applies in your baby's case.
If you have a breastfed infant, possibly diagnosed with reflux and possibly on medications, still having symptoms and reactions, even when you've tried a Total Elimination Diet (TED diet)	Most important now is to figure out what is causing your baby's reflux. This is my suggested order: Read Section 4.2 Cause Or Effect? (page 54), to help figure out the cause of your baby's reflux Read Section 5 Anatomy That Impacts Life (page 109) to understand your baby's natural digestive maturity Read Section 10 The Breastfeeding Protocol (page 199) and see if you're ready to do the elimination diet Understand my approach to food for babies in Section 8 Food for Babies (page 145).
If your baby is over 6 months, you've tried introducing solids and it has all gone tits-up	Read Section 5 Anatomy That Impacts Life (page 109) to understand your baby's natural digestive maturity Read Sections 11.3 Introducing Food (page 226) and 7.3 Reflux Flares With Solids (page 142) to see if this applies to your baby Download a food and symptom diary from https://www.thebabyrefluxlady.co.uk/book-reader and start recording to help identify patterns Read Section 8 Food for Babies (page 145), make a plan and change your baby's food to those they can more safely digest.
If you are considering medication for your baby	Read Section 4.9 Medical Solutions & Where To Find Them (page 78) Read Section 4.2 Cause Or Effect? (page 54), to help figure out the cause of your baby's reflux Using any new information, arm yourself with questions before you see your doctor about prescribing medication as a solution. Have a plan that you are happy with before accepting the medication. Know what you will do if it doesn't work, what your weaning plan is, how long baby will be on meds etc.

PART 1

THE COMMON EXPERIENCE OF REFLUX

1   FIRST STEPS

If your baby is struggling to settle, here are a few first steps that you should look at before jumping to conclusions about a reflux diagnosis. These questions will help you step through a simplified process so you understand what is going on for your baby, and find a way to remedy it sooner rather than later.

The questions you need to ask are presented in the order that you should answer them for a young baby. The sooner you can recognise anything awry, the quicker and better you can tackle it.

1. Do I have fair expectations of myself?
2. Do I have fair expectations of my baby?
3. What was our birth experience like?
4. Is my baby tired?
5. How is baby feeding?
6. What symptoms am I observing?
   a. Are they indicative of too much air being swallowed?
   b. Are they indicative of digestive discomfort?
7. How is my baby feeding?
8. What is in my baby's milk or food?

1.1   EXPECTATIONS OF YOURSELF

Becoming a parent is a life-changing experience. If you believe life can continue as it did before, you may need to have a little chat with yourself! The sooner you release yourself from all expectations of what parenthood is *supposed* to be like, the sooner you will give yourself greater freedom to best support yourself and your baby.

For the first few weeks, you and your baby are your number one priority. You must be gentle with both of these people. Remember that you have *given birth* to a human being. Regardless of how your baby has arrived into this world, you, your body, your baby and their body have all gone through a shock. Even if it was the most amazing birth ever, the sheer change required in your body to go from growing a baby to healing itself and perhaps feeding your child is massive.

This is the fourth trimester. This is *equally important for you* as your baby. Taking the Eastern philosophy of this time, allow your baby to still be "attached" to you and use this time as a gentle introduction of your baby into the world.

Your body has to go through enormous internal healing, sometimes external too. Your emotional and spiritual being must also accept great change, even if this is your second or more child. Give yourself time. Accept support. Even if it's not how you would do it...

1.2   EXPECTATIONS OF BABY

This question is a serious one. What do you want your baby to do? What are your expectations?

Know that baby really does nothing other than sleep and feed for the first few weeks. In the early days, your baby will naturally cling and want to be in your arms. Reflect on the dramatic change they have just experienced; baby's whole world is different, senses are awakening and being bombarded constantly. Baby will be looking to mummy for comfort. This is completely normal.

A friend of mine Nicky Woodhatch, director at Mummas and Beans, supports mums before and after birth. She often notices mums have unrealistic expectations of themselves and their babies. One of her most powerful tips is to "drop the pressure", which involves not putting so much pressure on yourself or your baby. "If you are finding your baby will only sleep on you, or with you, it is totally normal."[1] This also applies if

---

1 https://www.mummasandbeans.co.uk/blog/2017/3/21/thrive-not-survive-the-fourth-trimester

your baby is unsettled. Doing anything you can to reduce upset and crying will minimise the air they swallow and associated reflux symptoms.

1.3   WHAT WAS YOUR BABY'S BIRTH LIKE?

Birth is a traumatic experience, regardless of the birth you and your baby had. Your baby has gone from being curled up, safe and snug in a warm place, to being in a bright, open and intense environment. The process of getting there was also shocking.

Our bodies are incredible. Consider for a minute what our fragile and precious little baby goes through physically in being born. First, they are tucked up so tightly that they can barely wiggle their toes. Then, quite suddenly sometimes, they are squeezed firmly. Lots. And lots. Their head is squidged through a tiny space, what looks like zero space. This squeezing gets more and more intense.

If you have laboured, you know what this feels like from the outside. You know how strong those contractions can be. Imagine being physically squeezed on every side with that much intense pressure? I'm pretty sure it's not something you'd be keen to go do to your baby now, but this is what has just happened.

Sometimes the squeezing can last for hours. The bones of their skull physically move over each other during the birthing process in a vaginal delivery. Eventually, your baby is squeezed through the tightest of spaces and suddenly expelled by your body and into a dazzlingly bright place, where the feeling of everything is completely alien, unless it was a water birth.

The physical exertion on your baby's body distorts it. They twist and turn. They might be pulled and helped. All of this may result in their body not being 100% aligned with itself.

If a baby is born via caesarean section, it is nonetheless intense. Some may have gone through the squeezing, some may not. Yet, they are still ever-so-suddenly exposed to the outside world (however gentle the birth in our adult eyes) and lifted by the surgeon. While the physical trauma may not be as great, if it is an emergency C-section, baby may have been through much of the experience already.

In fact, everything other than a gentle and "easy" vaginal delivery can cause greater "trauma" to baby, if they are gently helped along by a midwife, if you were induced, if there was assistance by forceps or suction cup. All of it, can contribute to micro misalignments in your baby's structure that can cause reflux as a symptom.

Regardless of the way your baby was born, there is nothing but complete sensory overload when they arrive. This is where the infant craniosacral therapist, cranial osteopath or chiropractor comes in. These specialists have immense skills to support the natural realignment of your baby's body as well as yours. Any misalignment, however invisible to the external world, can introduce stressors within the body. Sometimes all your baby needs is a gentle realignment and many issues are improved or even resolved. Most therapists will see babies from 2 weeks. The power of realigning your baby's body can be incredible.

1.4   IS BABY TIRED?

Our newborn babies are like new toys. At least, our modern culture has us thinking of them as such. We are inundated with emails telling us the benefits of starting baby sign language from 2 weeks, swimming lessons at 6 weeks, baby sensory, yoga classes and play dates. We bring them out on walks every day. We chat to them; we sing to them.

"The Fourth Trimester is the school of thought that human babies are born at least 3 months too early. If we gave birth to them at 3, 4 or even 5 months they would be too big to deliver! We are one of the only species where our babies are born without the ability to do anything for themselves for a prolonged period of time."[2]

I fully understand the value in doing so many of these things. And yet, I believe there is something in giving your newborn time to be a baby. Time and space to rest, take in and process everything around them.

All of these activities may be fun and relaxing for you, but for your little one, time spent in a class with other babies and music and song and dancing and colours and textures... takes double the toll on them. All this new stimulation is interesting, yet there is a lot of effort required in processing it all.

Without control over their limbs, eyes or voice, crying is your baby's way of communicating. It's their only way of communicating with you... so listen carefully.

I have known a situation where a baby was so inconsolable and unsettled that the GP diagnosed reflux and prescribed drugs to resolve it. The drugs didn't work. Sleep did. This baby was not suffering from colic or reflux; he was overtired to the point of exhaustion.

If your baby is overtired, you must do whatever is necessary to help them sleep, even if it means sitting down on the sofa for an hour or more to allow them to sleep restfully, or carrying them in a carrier and going for a walk. Whatever it is, you must support your baby to sleep.

Sleep is the easiest place to start. And is important for all babies because *everything* is worse with tiredness.

To help you figure out if your baby is suffering from a lack of sleep, ask these questions:

- How long has baby been awake? If it has been more than 2 hours, chances are baby needs a rest.

---

2 https://www.mummasandbeans.co.uk/blog/2017/3/21/thrive-not-survive-the-fourth-trimester

- Does holding baby close enough to stop them flailing their arms help them to settle?

- Does your baby stop crying to breathe, or snooze for a minute or two? A baby in pain will not stop crying.

- Is baby happiest when upright? Does baby appear to have a pattern of disliking lying down? If this dislike is a strong objection to lying down and baby appears to be considerably uncomfortable, this is a clear sign that some reflux could be irritating them.

Do everything in your power to make sure your baby is rested.

1.5   How is Baby Feeding?

Note: For All babies with feeding discomfort, please check out the updated Oral Play and Tongue Tie online course which explores oral function in much greater detail than is available in this book.
www.thebabyrefluxlady.co.uk/book-reader

If your baby is swallowing too much air, they will inevitably show signs of colic or reflux. When this happens and baby is "drinking" too much air, there is little that alternate milks or medication can do.

I believe *every* baby should be assessed for a tongue-tie within their first 2 or 3 days of life. If feeding problems continue or arise after 2 to 8 weeks old, baby should be reassessed. Speaking from personal experience, the development of the mouth and tongue in the first few weeks can bring a previously unidentifiable tongue-tie into play. Regardless of whether baby is breast- or bottle-fed, a tongue-tie, if present, can cause longer-term problems and impacts that are much more easily dealt with in the early days.

The only people properly qualified to assess for a tongue-tie are International Board Certified Lactation Consultants[3] (IBCLC), Tongue Tie Practitioners (UK), or a specialist paediatric speech therapist.

I recommend that *every* baby sees a lactation consultant, even if you are bottle-feeding. While many breastfeeding counsellors may have the knowledge and experience to correctly assess a tongue-tie, a posterior tongue-tie can be easily missed. I believe IBCLCs have the knowledge and capability to assess the latch your baby has on the breast or bottle, and can determine how much air baby is drinking when feeding. Your health visitor, GP, and paediatric consultants rarely have the skills required to assess this.

Our paediatric consultant told me that Daffodil did not have a tongue-tie and prescribed her some strong reflux medication. Later, I had her tongue-tie resolved, which immediately changed our lives.

You can watch out for key signs yourself. Your baby's latch may not be as good as it could be if *any* of the following are true. In these circumstances, a consultation for latch or tongue-tie is crucial.

- Is there any milk leaking or spilling from their mouth as they drink?
- Do they gulp, choke or gag when drinking?
- Can you hear them gulping?
- Can you hear milk sloshing in their tummy?
- Do they bob on and off the breast?
- Do they try to adjust their latch on their bottle?
- Do they appear to be frustrated when feeding?
- Do they make a clicking sound when feeding?

---

3 From this point forward, when I mention lactation consultants, I mean International Board Certified Lactation Consultants. This qualification is different from a breastfeeding counsellor's.

If you observe any of these signs, spend at least half an hour after a feed winding your baby. It is much easier to release wind upwards than suffer the pain and discomfort of additional air moving through the gut.

Furthermore, if your baby is bottle-fed and drinking too much air, try the Medela Calma bottle and teat. http://geni.us/Medela

See Section 4.3 Tongue-Tie & Reflux (page 60) for more detail on tongue-tie and latch.

1.6   HOW MUCH IS BABY FEEDING?

Another consideration is the volume of milk your baby is drinking. If there is a lot of spit-up, reduce the volume of your baby's feeds. Think of your baby's tummy as a full juice carton with a straw. If it is full, then lying it down or squeezing it will cause it to overflow. Baby's tummy is much the same in response to tummy contractions.

When the pressure in the stomach is higher than the pressure in the oesophagus, the stomach contents can get forced out quite easily. One contributing factor to the pressure in the stomach is the volume of milk in it.

During the first few days of life, your baby's stomach cannot stretch or increase in volume in the way a more mature stomach can. This was observed in 1920[4]. This is important to understand because in the early days, there lack of stomach elasticity means baby really does need small and frequent feeds, hence why colostrum is so nutritionally dense and is present for the first few days post partum.

I believe that we should adopt a much more natural approach to milk and food quantity for our children to support them in the way that they were designed. Overfeeding will not just potentially cause digestive discomfort, reflux and colic[5]; it can lead to obesity in our infants. It is well-documented that higher levels of protein in formula milks versus breastmilk result in children becoming obese[6].

---

4 "Observations on the capacity of the stomach in the first ten days of postnatal life.", R. Scammon, L O'Doyle, American Journal of Dis Child 1920. http://bit.ly/BRLNewbornStomach
5 https://www.kidspot.com.au/baby/feeding/bottle-feeding/the-dangers-of-overfeeding-your-bottlefed-baby/news-story/52634fe00f5f185bab9dfbcb0d26e961
6 Campbell KJ, Abbott G, Zheng M, McNaughton SA. Early Life Protein Intake: Food Sources, Correlates, and Tracking across the First 5 Years of Life. J Acad Nutr Diet. 2017 Aug; 117(8):1188-1197.e1. doi: 10.1016/j.jand.2017.03.016. Epub 2017 May 17. PubMed PMID: 28527745.
https://www.ncbi.nlm.nih.gov/pubmed/28527745

If your baby is spitting up after every meal, do smaller feeds and more frequently[7]. If you are concerned that baby is spitting up everything, not passing stools and not weeing enough, visit you GP to speak about pyloric stenosis.

1.7   Is There Something In Baby's Food?

1.7.1   Breastfeeding

If baby is breastfeeding and showing signs of significant discomfort, but not appearing to drink too much air, there may be something in your breastmilk that baby cannot digest fully. There are many reasons why this may happen. While this book does not deal with the extensive reasons for this, we will cover how to change your diet to minimise the irritants to your baby. See Section 10 The Breastfeeding Protocol (page 199) for more information.

1.7.2   Formula-Fed Infants

Like with breastmilk, formula may not agree with your little baby's naturally immature yet perfectly healthy digestive system. So many ingredients of formula can trigger a reaction. Every baby is different and so the answer to this problem may be different for every baby.

Be careful not to jump straight to the conclusion that your baby has cow's milk protein allergy (CMPA) or a lactose intolerance. First, make sure that baby's latch is 100%. Then, if you see some of the following symptoms, there may be an allergy or intolerance at play.

Any one of these symptoms, alone, does not constitute a diagnosis; nor should you rely on the information in this book alone for diagnosing health issues with your child. For more detail about trying to figure out what is going on for your baby, read Section 3 Colic, Reflux, Allergy or Intolerance? (page 30). If you see two or more of the below symptoms

---

7   https://www.nice.org.uk/guidance/ng1/resources/gastrooesophageal-reflux-disease-in-children-and-young-people-diagnosis-and-management-51035086789 Page 20

consistently, it is worth starting to explore different milks. Use Section 6 What's In Baby's Milk? (page 125) to help your decision about what you should try next and how.

Without any of the "too much air" symptoms above, your baby experiences:

- Stomach issues like:
    o   Abdominal distension
    o   Bloating
    o   Rock hard tummy
- Respiratory issues[8] that are not improving after 7 days like:
    o   Runny nose
    o   Congestion
    o   Cough
    o   Hives
    o   Sleep apnoea
- Skin rashes, hives, rosacea or eczema
- Constipation or diarrhoea
- Mucus in poo
- Green poo
- Offensive odour from poo

1.7.3   BABIES ON SOLIDS

Many babies experience reflux flare-ups when solids are introduced. The most common answer to this is increasing medication dosage. At this point, the cause of the flare-ups is not medication-related, but food-related. Read Section 5 Anatomy That Impacts Life (page 109) and Section 8 Food for Babies (page 145) to fully understand how food interacts with your baby's system.

---

8 If any of the respiratory issues appear with a fever, consult your GP immediately.

When weaning or introducing solids, take it slowly. There is a mind-shift to be made between what society suggests and what may be best for your baby. Be gentle. You will be rewarded.

2   YOU'VE HAD A BABY! NOW WHAT?

Congratulations! You are a parent! You want to give your child the best start in life, I'm sure. You will do anything to support your little one in their growth and development. You want them to sail through life as easily and carefree as possible.

You are your child's primary teacher and carer. You will give them the foundation for everything they learn, live, see, choose. What you do over the first 16 years of your child's life will influence almost everything they do for the rest of their life. You will instil beliefs and values, show them how to make choices independently. You will teach them how to feel and react. You will give them the foundation for their health. Sure, your child will make their own choices from an early age; *you* supply the framework for *how* those choices happen.

From a health perspective, there are two elements to long-term strong health – genetics and environment. Genetics are the part we cannot change, but that doesn't matter because environment accounts for about 80% of health, as I have discovered. Genetics make us more prone to develop different types of diseases later in life, but I am convinced that we can overcome shortfalls in our genetic make-up to maximise our own health and live a long and healthy life. What's more, I believe this applies to 95% of the population or more.

Knowing that, are you willing to learn about how food influences your child's body? Do you want to do the best for them? Do you want them to have exceptional health and be resistant to illness? It all starts now. You can give your child one of the greatest gifts: a foundation for good health.

To understand the journey to life-long health, we must understand how babies are different to adults, how they develop and mature, and how the food they eat can help or hinder them. Along with this understanding, we must remember that until the age of 5, children have an extremely high propensity to learn and develop, to amaze and surprise us, to develop in untold ways. This is therefore the right time to encourage them to be self-aware, knowing how food impacts their bodies. Digestion and growth are no different to any other area of their self-awareness.

While a proportion of their growth and capacity is governed by genetics, for the majority of children, environment trumps genes. Keep this in mind as you teach them. Give your child the best start in life.

IMPORTANT! *Do not* force your child to finish everything on their plate. Instead, negotiate another few forkfuls. Tell them there are no snacks if they haven't eaten their meal and enforce this rule. This is all you need do.

2.1   What If Baby Just Won't Settle?

For some babies, like my first daughter Sunflower, you know from the first 24 hours that something is not quite right. For me, this was walking the wards all night long on my own because she wouldn't stop crying, unless she was on my boob. And that hurt. A lot! I knew she couldn't stay there all night too. For other newborns, it might be a gradual progression to sleepless nights after a few days or weeks.

The reality is, though, if you have a baby who will not settle, you will know about it. Chances are baby is happiest on your boob or shoulder. And yep, you guessed it. There's a strong preference for mummy's shoulder above anyone else's.

You may experience baby crying a lot, or a lot at night. Maybe your elders and peers are telling you about the "witching hours" – those hours between 7pm and 11pm when babies just cry. Maybe you've had at least 3 hours of inconsolable crying for at least 3 days a week for at least 3 weeks, in which case someone else will tell you "it's just colic" and that baby will grow out of it.

In truth, I don't believe in colic, and I don't believe in the witching hours. I have come to realise they are catch-all terms for what the medical profession doesn't understand. Either that or terms coined to allow Western parents the convenience of life they were used to before baby and ignore the fundamental fourth trimester. That includes overlooking baby's digestive immaturity and the real reasons they may be unsettled.

Regardless of what people are telling you, you still feel something is wrong. And there *is* action you can take. If you have a baby who is constantly crying and won't settle, here are my suggestions on what do, how to do it and why each step is important.

2.2   WHAT'S CAUSING BABY'S DISCOMFORT?

The very first step to take is listening to your baby's cry, which is their only way of communicating with you right now. It's your job to figure out what your little one is trying to tell you. There are a number of practitioners who can help you interpret your baby's cry's, I loved Tracy Hogg, The Baby Whisper's fabulous explanations of how baby is communicating. I could tell what my baby was 'saying' from about 3 weeks of age. You can find her explanations detailed in her book Secrets of the Baby Whisperer. (http://geni.us/BabyWhisperer)

2.2.1   THE ASSISTED METHOD

I have developed a short mini-course summarising this information, with an interactive quiz to help you work out what is likely going on for your baby. You can access that at this link (http://geni.us/RefluxCause). As part of the e-course I host regular live Q&A sessions to provide you additional help.

2.2.2   THE DIY METHOD

Here's how to apply this information yourself in a series of steps.

STEP 1

Know that reflux is normal. Ask yourself: is baby in pain because of reflux or something else? Learn to interpret your baby's cries, because baby has different cries depending on what is going on. Listen carefully and patiently. Refer to a crying expert to try and interpret what your baby is saying.

STEP 2

Is your baby tired? Are they sleeping enough for their age? If they are tired do *everything* in your power to help them sleep, a baby who gets their sleep will be easier for everyone to deal with

STEP 3

Ask yourself: does baby suffer from any of the common symptoms? Figure 1 overleaf outlines the most common symptoms reported by parents of unsettled babies (reflux, colic and/or CMPA).

STEP 4

While many of these symptoms are often described as reflux symptoms, I believe they can point us toward the *cause* of the reflux. See Section 4.1 When Reflux Is a Problem (page 47) to learn how to read the symptoms you are observing so you can better understand where the root of your baby's symptoms might be.

STEP 5

Keep a food and symptom diary for a few days. Observe and record everything so that you can see and measure any changes that might happen. I cannot stress enough the importance of doing this first, because if you're a tired mum, making reasonable judgements from memory from week to week is difficult.

You can download a free food and symptom diary template at https://www.thebabyrefluxlady.co.uk/book-reader.

Most Common Symptoms exhibited

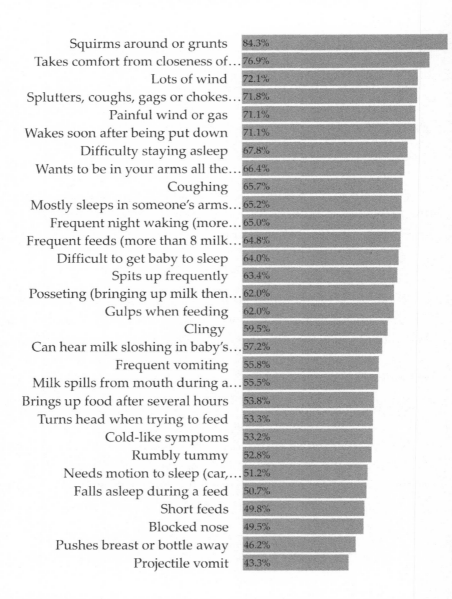

Symptom	Percentage
Squirms around or grunts	84.3%
Takes comfort from closeness of...	76.9%
Lots of wind	72.1%
Splutters, coughs, gags or chokes...	71.8%
Painful wind or gas	71.1%
Wakes soon after being put down	71.1%
Difficulty staying asleep	67.8%
Wants to be in your arms all the...	66.4%
Coughing	65.7%
Mostly sleeps in someone's arms...	65.2%
Frequent night waking (more...	65.0%
Frequent feeds (more than 8 milk...	64.8%
Difficult to get baby to sleep	64.0%
Spits up frequently	63.4%
Posseting (bringing up milk then...	62.0%
Gulps when feeding	62.0%
Clingy	59.5%
Can hear milk sloshing in baby's...	57.2%
Frequent vomiting	55.8%
Milk spills from mouth during a...	55.5%
Brings up food after several hours	53.8%
Turns head when trying to feed	53.3%
Cold-like symptoms	53.2%
Rumbly tummy	52.8%
Needs motion to sleep (car,...	51.2%
Falls asleep during a feed	50.7%
Short feeds	49.8%
Blocked nose	49.5%
Pushes breast or bottle away	46.2%
Projectile vomit	43.3%

Figure 1 details the most common symptoms from my survey (data taken from my Reflux Survey with 1196 unique respondents). The percentages are the proportion of babies who experienced each particular symptom, as observed by their parents.

STEP 6

If baby is at least 2 weeks old, bring them to see a craniosacral osteopath or chiropractor. We forget that the birthing process is a massive physical ordeal for baby's body. They, as well as mum, go through some massive physical strains.

Baby's skull is designed to move, for the bones to overlap each other during birth. If your baby's body is not realigned shortly after birth, the invisible misalignments can introduce stress and discomfort.

A therapist who has specialist training in paediatrics can adjust your baby and help their body settle into their new life. This alone can result in massive change for baby's latch, sleep and digestive system function. Repeat treatments may be required to make sure the adjustments "stick" and become the new "normal" position, and to support your baby's body as it goes through such rapid growth and development.

STEP 7

Establish the non-medical actions you can take first to rule out other issues that might be going on:

a) Has baby got a good sleep routine? If not, spend a few days getting baby rested, regardless of where this has to be, in the buggy, in a carrier, on your shoulder. Concentrate on ruling out any issues that might be due to overtiredness alone.

b) How much is your baby drinking in one go? Is the milk too much for their stomach to cope with? If so, it has nowhere to go but up and out.

Have you winded your baby properly? This can help if your baby is drinking too much air because of any latch problems or potential tongue-tie. It can reduce reflux simply by removing air effectively from the stomach, because what goes in must come out.

c) Get baby checked for a tongue-tie. If baby has a tongue-tie, they will not be able to remove milk from the breast properly and will swallow air, as well as have long and/or very frequent feeds.

d) Consult a lactation consultant to have your baby's latch checked. If baby is not latching perfectly, then they will be swallowing air as well as milk, and not be removing milk as effectively as possible from the breast.

e) If baby is bottle-fed, check that their latch on the teat is perfect. If you see spilling or dribbling from baby's mouth while feeding, they aren't forming a full seal and air will be getting in too. Try a range of bottle teats to see if you can minimise air intake. My favourite is the Medela Calma teat because it requires baby to suck before removing air from the bottle http://geni.us/Medela

Pay attention to feeding all the time, but especially for night-time feeds to reduce air intake. Focus on a better latch. Sit baby upright a little. Hold baby upright for 30 minutes after a feed to let gravity help digestion.

f) Your baby might be sensitive to something in your breastmilk. I recommend eliminating all dairy and all soy products (including most dark chocolate containing soy-derived emulsifier), eggs, wheat and nuts. This may sound like a big ask, but try it for 2 weeks and see if there's a difference. Then you can reintroduce foods one at a time. A massive effort now could result in an amazing outcome much sooner. You could save yourself 6 months of sleep loss and everything else that goes with it.

g) Give baby a tummy massage after bath and before bedtime to boost their little digestive system. You can also try reflexology (foot massage) to support digestion and the movement of air through the body.

h) If your baby is spitting up a lot, then try reducing the volume of milk in any one feed.

If these don't give any relief at all, then it is time to see your GP and bring all the information with you of what you have tried. This gives you a strong basis from the start. Plus, if you've got your food and symptom diary with you, you **know** you won't forget to describe exactly how much anguish you're going through.

2.3   WHERE DO I GET ADVICE?

This is a great question! Most parents assume that their GP is the first port of call. If not the GP, perhaps the health visitor. However, in the UK, your midwife will usually be the first point of contact until baby is 6 weeks old; after the midwife has released you from their care, you are under the care of your GP. The problem is none of these professionals are qualified in any way, shape or form to advise you on food *unless* they have an additional qualification in nutrition or dietetics. And chances are they haven't had time to read the research available.

One of the most shocking discoveries I made while writing this book is that it takes 17 years for bona fide research to make its way into general practice. 17 years! So everything that is being published now, stuff that is being talked about in the media, stuff about food that we see in 'reality' type TV programmes, and stuff that is currently being studied in research facilities and **known** to be the best advice available, none of that will come through your health professional for another 17 years! Until your child is an adult! That's the same age as people are allowed to vote in some countries! That's why I stopped seeking advice about food from my GP. That's also why I stopped discussing any of my food and nutritional opinions with my GP.

What did I do instead? When Sunflower decided to stop breastfeeding at 12 months, she still needed additional nutrition from a milk that she wasn't going to get from food. Her intolerances went further than dairy; she wasn't able to drink so-called "normal" brands of milk alternatives due to the additives in them. I consulted a dietician and had honest conversations with her. However, I felt I couldn't get her personal opinion on my concerns and questions; she worked for the NHS, which doesn't allow professionals to act outside the rules they generally deem to be "right", regardless of updated evidence. The system is shocking but that's another hobby horse!

Did you know GPs get **less than 1 week**[9] of nutritional training in their entire 7 years of study, relating to all the patients they may encounter? In fact, nutrition, diet and food are not even listed on the subjects for students at either Oxford or Cambridge medical schools in the UK at the time of writing. If they are studied, it appears these subjects are buried somewhere as a minor topic.

A dietician will have studied for 3 years, plus another year in clinical practice, and has to register with the Health and Care Professions Council (HCPC). I know where I would prefer to get dietary advice.

So why do you need this book if you could get all your answers from seeing a dietician? Well, because they are not necessarily qualified to talk about food intolerances either! In fact, there is no specialist study or profession for the management of food intolerances. Only for allergies.

Typically, your GP will manage symptoms, but will not uncover the root cause that could make the problem go away. I prefer to discover the cause and avoid whatever causes symptoms to occur, rather than take medication, drugs or prescriptions that could cause long-term harm. In short, I choose to help my child grow properly.

---

9 The amount of time dedicated to food, diet and nutrition varies from one medical school to the next, but in no school is it taught as a major subject to everyone studying medicine.

What does that leave us with? Facebook. Funnily enough, *you are not alone* if you're currently getting all your information from groups on social media! Many have been through this before. Indeed, you'll be surprised how many parents are going through it right now. One of the greatest gifts I can give you is the knowledge that *you are not alone*, and you don't have to do it on your own. There are many support forums on Facebook, and other places online, for your specific situation. You can find my group at www.fb.com/groups/babyrefluxlady . Feel free to come and join us there for daily support.

3   COLIC, REFLUX, ALLERGY OR INTOLERANCE?

There is a massive list of health conditions with which healthy infants and children are diagnosed. Many of these, I understand, are the result of either excessive strain on their digestive systems or being fed the wrong food completely. In my opinion, medication should be used only as a last resort, because there is far too much use of prescription drugs in young babies and infants. In Section 3, we'll be looking at how to tell whether your baby's unsettledness is about colic, reflux, allergy or intolerance, including the importance of managing these correctly, the impact they have on parents, sleep, relationships, communication and the rest of the family.

As I will go on to outline in Section 5 Anatomy That Impacts Life (page 109), babies are born underdeveloped compared to an adult. The fact we have stages in life – from infancy, childhood, adolescence into adulthood – is a sign that we need to acknowledge a baby's relative underdevelopment. We observe the physical and emotional changes that happen to a person throughout these stages in life, but the ability of the digestive system is completely overlooked. We look only at the nutritional requirements to fuel massive growth and change and, as a society, tend to ignore or perhaps fail to think about the ability of the body's digestive system and its needs.

3.1   SYMPTOMS: WHAT TO LOOK FOR

"You are what you eat" became a popular phrase some years ago. To an extent, this is true, but the phrase is misunderstood. What we put into our bodies is vital to their behaviour, growth, development and emotions. We must understand how the body uses different types of food.

If you feel that your baby is unhappy all the time except when hungry, you might be able to do something about it. If you know what to look for, you can interpret the signs and understand how to help.

While there is never a complete list of all symptoms for all babies, this is comprehensive and a good place to start. These symptoms are listed in relation to when you might observe them. After this list, you will find groupings of symptoms into likely causes and, importantly, what action you can take to remedy your baby's discomfort or unease.

There is a place for medication for babies, but as a last resort. In my view, this option is just one short of surgery. If there are actions we can take to support baby's *natural growth and development*, that's what we should do first.

You can use this list to assess your baby's behaviour, and give yourself the confidence that what you are observing is not "just normal behaviour". I hope to help you trust yourself. Some of these symptoms are indicative of reflux, some of tiredness, others of latch issues. I want you to understand, too, that in almost all of these cases, there is an underlying *cause* of the symptom and you can do something.

Have a read and record any symptoms you observe in your baby, even score them from 1-10 for severity or frequency.

FEEDING

- Frequent feeds (more than 8 times per day after the first 4 weeks)
- Short feeds
- Falling asleep during a feed (at nap- and bed-time is fine; if most feeds, it could be a problem)
- Frequent refusal to feed
- Pushing breast or bottle away
- Turning head when trying to feed
- Tugging at the breast during a feed
- Milk spills from mouth during a feed
- Milk comes back up through nose
- Posseting (bringing up milk then swallowing it again)
- Spluttering, coughing, gagging or choking during a feed

- Gulping when feeding
- Clawing at face or breast when feeding
- Hitting when feeding
- Bobbing on and off the breast during a feed
- Hearing milk sloshing in baby's tummy
- Spitting up frequently

AFTER FEEDING

- Projectile vomit
- Frequent vomiting
- Green or yellow vomiting
- Vomit has blood in it*
- Choking or blue spells**
- Bringing up food after several hours
- Always bringing up most milk after 30 to 90 minutes, and always hungry***
- Squirming around or grunting

SLEEP

- Frequent night waking (more than twice a night from 8 weeks)
- Sleep apnoea (stops breathing for a period)**
- Mostly sleeping in someone's arms or on shoulder
- Difficulty getting baby to sleep
- Waking soon after being put down
- Difficulty staying asleep
- Needing motion to sleep (car, bouncing, buggy)
- Restless sleep

RESPIRATORY

- Coughing
- Blocked nose

- Runny nose
- Cold-like symptoms
- Difficulty breathing (any time of the day or night)**
- Face goes blue**
- Constant or recurring infections
- Wheezing**
- Stridor (high-pitched wheezing)**

DIGESTIVE SYSTEM

- Acidic breath
- Smelly breath
- Rumbly tummy
- Rock hard tummy
- Tender tummy
- Swollen tummy
- Bloated abdomen (any time of the day or night)
- Diarrhoea
- Constipation
- Mucus in poo
- Blood in poo*
- Green poo
- Black, foul-smelling poo*
- Lots of wind
- Painful wind or gas
- Itchy bottom

GENERAL

- Hiccoughing frequently
- Sneezing frequently
- Eczema
- Spots or rashes
- Disliking lying down

- Disliking having nappy changed
- Clingy, wanting to be in arms
- Needing to be close to mum all the time
- Lethargy*
- Inexplicable high temperature (37.5C or more)*
- Poor weight gain
- Weight loss*
- Failure to thrive
- Excessive weight gain
- Large weight fluctuations*
- Arching of back
- Stretching neck
- Drawing legs up to tummy
- Constant crying
- Excessive crying
- High-pitched crying
- Painful crying
- Screaming
- Unsettled or unhappy baby
- Irritability
- Difficulty establishing a routine
- Difficulty predicting what baby will want/need
- Dark marks under eyes
- Hives
- General restlessness
- Constant infections
- Muscle pain in arms and/or legs
- Jerky or dystonic head and neck movements (Sandifer's Syndrome)*

BEHAVIOURAL

- Temper tantrums

- Excessive whining
- Excessive screaming
- Excessive clinginess
- Hyperactivity
- Aggression
  - Biting
  - Hitting
  - Spitting
  - Pinching
  - Punching
  - Kicking
- Repetition of speech
- Non-stop, senseless talk
- Food cravings
- Reluctance to smile
- Excessive fatigue
- Depression
- Refusal to stay dressed
- Refusal to be touched
- Desire to hide in darkness

Many of the symptoms above can be normal, or can occur to any baby in response to a particular stimulus, including overtiredness, stress, change, emotions, seasons, colds and various other external inputs. How do we know if it's down to a food intolerance or an allergy? We will go on to explore this question, but first, a word of warning about certain symptoms.

All of the asterisk-marked symptoms should be treated as a red flag. These require quick, even immediate medical attention.

* Any indication of blood requires investigation. Consult your GP immediately. Request an initial phone conversation (which can often be quicker than waiting for an appointment).

** Any indication of difficulty breathing should be checked immediately as an A&E emergency. It may be that your baby has enlarged adenoids (soft tissue at the back of the nose) or something relatively benign and will be okay. However, as breath is required for life, there is zero point in taking any risks.

*** This can be an indication of pyloric stenosis. Typically appearing at around 6 weeks, it requires immediate attention and surgery to be rectified.

3.2   RED FLAG SYMPTOMS

There are a number of symptoms that indicate something else going on rather than reflux. According to the UK's National Institute for Health and Care Excellence (NICE), if your baby has regurgitation and vomiting plus any of the red flag symptoms, then it may be something other than GORD (so-called gastro-oesophageal reflux disease, or GERD in the US) and your baby requires primary care management, hospital admission or specialist referral depending on clinical judgement. These red flag symptoms[10] are as follows:

- Frequent, forceful (projectile) vomiting – suggests hypertrophic pyloric stenosis in infants up to 2 months old.
- Bile-stained (green or yellow-green) vomit – suggests intestinal obstruction.
- Abdominal distension, tenderness, or palpable mass – suggests intestinal obstruction or another acute surgical condition.
- Haematemesis (blood in vomit) except for swallowed blood, for example, following a nosebleed or ingested blood from a cracked nipple in some breastfed infants – suggests an important and potentially serious bleed from the oesophagus, stomach, or upper gut.

---

10 https://cks.nice.org.uk/gord-in-children#!diagnosissub:2

- Bulging fontanelle ('soft spot') or altered responsiveness (for example, lethargy or irritability) – suggests raised intracranial pressure (caused by meningitis, for example).

- Rapidly increasing head circumference (more than 1cm each week); persistent morning headache and vomiting worse in the morning – suggests raised intracranial pressure (caused by hydrocephalus, also known as 'water on the brain', or a brain tumour, for example).

- Blood in the stool – suggests a variety of conditions, including bacterial gastroenteritis, infant cow's milk protein allergy.

- Chronic diarrhoea – suggests cow's milk protein allergy.

- With, or at high risk of, atopy (for example, atopic dermatitis, asthma, eczema, allergic rhinitis).

- Symptoms of a urinary tract infection, for example dysuria (difficulty passing urine).

- Appearing unwell or fever – suggests infection.

- Onset of regurgitation and/or vomiting after 6 months of age or persisting after 1 year of age – suggests a cause other than reflux, for example, urinary tract infection.

If your baby presents with any of the above, consult your GP immediately. If you are dissatisfied with their response, then request a different GP or a straight referral to an allergist (for example, if you suspect CMPA).

If you ever have cause for immediate concern, do not hesitate to visit your A&E unit.

3.3   COLIC

The UK NHS states, "Colic is the name for excessive, frequent crying in a baby who appears to be otherwise healthy [...] the problem will eventually pass and is usually nothing to worry about."[11]

Personally, I don't believe in the way Western medicine defines "colic". Colic is a term commonly used by modern medicine to accommodate a convenient lifestyle, one where we don't have to make dietary changes for the benefit of our babies.

From my investigations, I suggest there is a reason for colic: digestive upset. In horses, colic is understood to be a very serious condition. All horse owners understand it so well that they take active steps to avoid it because a horse cannot vomit, so it can be a real matter of life and death. Thankfully, it is not so serious in babies, but I highlight this because we *can do something about it*. We can alter our diet, or that of our baby, and ease the discomfort in the digestive system.

Medical descriptions for recognising colic are correct – babies cry inconsolably until they get relief, typically after 3 hours of crying, with intermittent periods of settling in parents' arms, bouncing or swaying. Often after 5-10 minutes of being settled, with mum or dad still in bouncing mode, something else happens and baby is in pain again. After hours of crying baby will pass gas, lots of it, and will cry harder passing the gas. Eventually, baby will settle.

The medical definition of colic symptoms includes at least 3 hours of crying, 3 nights a week, for 3 weeks or more. This is useless information to anyone. Professionals go on to say that some infant drops, such as enzyme drops or gripe water, help settle colic. However, colicky babies are in *genuine digestive pain or discomfort*. Western medicine gives little or no recognition to digestive immaturity in young babies. Advice says to put up with it and baby will grow out of it. What is really happening when a baby

---

11 http://www.nhs.uk/conditions/Colic/Pages/Introduction.aspx

"grows out of" colic is that baby's digestive system matures a bit to be able to digest the foods that have been irritating them. But why should they put up with the pain when it is avoidable? That's right. I believe the accumulation of gas in baby's gut causes discomfort and pain until the gas has passed; and furthermore, that this gas build-up and the resulting **pain is avoidable**.

If, in most cases, "gas" is trapped in baby's system causing pain and colicky behaviour, I say there is a reason... a cause. The trick is to find out what each baby's specific cause is and deal with the root of the problem. Causes can be multiple and from a vast range.

Babies are born with an immature digestive system. Breastfeeding mums are not advised to modify diet to reflect what newborn infants can digest. Many professionals argue that food does not pass into breastmilk, but will readily agree that babies can be allergic to cow's milk proteins passed through the breastmilk. This contradiction leads me to believe that any substance in a mother's bloodstream has the potential to pass the blood-milk barrier and so pass into baby's digestive system.

And it's not just a hunch. Literature by La Leche League states, "When someone takes medication or eats food, the substance is usually broken down by the digestive tract and then molecule-sized components of the substance are absorbed into the blood. When these molecules get to the capillaries near the breast tissue, they move through the cells that line the alveoli and into the milk, a process known as diffusion."[12] By this mechanism, substances can pass into breastmilk. And each new substance has the potential to irritate a baby's immature gut.

See Section 9 Foundations of Change (page 186) for using diet and eating habits to positively influence your baby's colic.

My private clients see and believe the direct link between the food they eat and their baby's temperament, comfort and behaviour. For example, if

---

12 http://www.lalecheleague.org/nb/nbmarapr05p44.html

there is a suspicion of dairy intolerance, cutting out dairy and soy often gives some positive changes. When we take it further and cut out the foods that baby's immature digestive system cannot break down, those foods that are likely to ferment, we get even greater positive benefits. The details of how to do this for yourself are outlined in Section 9 Foundations of Change (page 186).

3.4   REFLUX & SILENT REFLUX

When my baby wouldn't sleep, I couldn't figure it out. When she lost weight, I couldn't figure it out. When she still wouldn't sleep, I still couldn't figure it out. And when my baby repeatedly came back to my breast as the happiest place in the world for her, I couldn't not let her have it.

Eventually, I realised it was reflux of the silent type (no vomiting). She was about 5½ months old by then and I figured it out, finally, by way of a 3am Dr Google diagnosis. The medical answer that came, the answer from a highly-paid consultant, was to give her a daily dose of prescription drug domperidone, a drug for which the side effects include: dry mouth, abdominal cramps, diarrhoea, nausea, rash, itching, and hives.

Okay, so I have a question... Why on earth would I give my daughter a medication that puts undue strain on her infantile liver? *Surely, there must be another way.* And there was, though not an immediately obvious one. My understanding of reflux at the time, from everything I'd read, was that there was no suggestion of dairy being a potential irritant. But my life and my understanding were about to change radically...

3.4.1   WHAT IS REFLUX?

Ever met a "happy spitter"? Or met a mother who always has a muslin draped over her shoulder but baby is the happiest child on the planet? You see, reflux, lots of posseting and vomiting milk, is often totally normal. It only becomes a problem if it is causing pain or discomfort for your baby.

As part of digestive development, the lower oesophageal sphincter (LOS/LES in the US) muscle that shuts off the oesophagus (food pipe) from the stomach is naturally weaker in infants than in older children and adults. It will strengthen naturally with growth. Due to the developmental stage of a baby's digestive system at birth, contents of the stomach can return up through the LOS. In many cases, this does not cause a problem for baby. Yet many babies are being diagnosed with reflux or silent reflux, when reflux is completely normal, not a diagnosis.

Gastro-oesophageal reflux (simply referred to as *reflux*) is when the contents of the stomach regurgitate up into the oesophagus. Reflux is when the LOS is not strong enough to keep the contents of the stomach from coming back up. This is more a sign of the immaturity of a baby's digestive system than a health issue. Most babies grow out of reflux by 12 months. It is a maturity issue. ***Reflux in babies does not have the same origin as reflux in adults, and so it should be managed differently.***

Normal processes in the body continue, so once food arrives in the stomach, the stomach starts to churn the food. At about 30 to 90 minutes after this churning process starts, there is a strong contraction of the stomach designed to push food through the lower sphincter muscle and on into the small intestine. In babies with a weaker upper sphincter muscle, this can cause the food to be pushed back up into the oesophagus too. When this happens, the milk or food has been mixed with stomach acid, which can burn the lining of the oesophagus and the throat depending on how far the regurgitation reaches.

In many children, vomiting, posseting (small amounts of milk regurgitation), projectile vomiting is an indicator of potential reflux. However, there are some children who never vomit yet still suffer from reflux. This is called *silent reflux* and is often missed or diagnosed as colic because of its silent nature, when there is actually something else going on.

3.5   ALLERGIES & INTOLERANCES

Allergies and food intolerances are not as difficult to spot as you might think. The trick is to be observant of your child and critique what has happened so far. If you feel like you've tried so many things, and nothing has really changed, it's time to take it back to basics. If your child repeatedly has three of the symptoms listed in 3.1 Symptoms: What To Look For (page 30) constantly, it is highly likely that they are experiencing an irritation from an external stimulus. This stimulus is as constant as the symptoms so there are a few questions to ask yourself:

1. Does your child suffer simultaneously from two or more of the symptoms listed overleaf, on a regular basis and for prolonged periods of time? (Example: cold-like symptoms that don't improve over the course of a few weeks.)
2. Do your child's symptoms change with the seasons?
3. Does your child improve when they are in a different place for a few days? (Example: better on holidays, at grandparents' house, because this could indicate an intolerance or allergy to something in the environment)

    or

    Are your child's symptoms constant regardless of location? This could indicate something that is constant in their life, so not environmentally driven, but more towards foods.

If you answer 'yes' to any of the above, then it is highly likely that your child's body is responding to an external stimulus. The next step is to start a detailed food and symptom diary, including environmental information if you think it may be relevant.

For example, when you go swimming, baby's behaviour is noticeably out of character for a few hours afterwards. You recognise this is a regular pattern. This could be highly indicative of your baby being exposed to too much chlorine, which is linked to "higher risk of bronchiolitis, with ensuing increased risks of asthma and allergic sensitisation".[13]

Symptoms that are likely to indicate an allergic response or intolerance include:

DIGESTIVE SYSTEM

- Vomiting (without fever)
- Choking or blue spells
- Bringing up food after several hours
- Squirming around or grunting
- Rock hard tummy
- Tender tummy
- Swollen tummy
- Bloated abdomen (any time of the day or night)
- Diarrhoea or constipation
- Mucus in poo
- Green poo
- Black in poo (except after eating a banana)
- Lots of wind
- Painful wind or gas
- Itchy bottom

SLEEP

- Restless sleep
- Snoring
- Sleep apnoea (breathing stops for a period)
- Difficulty staying asleep

---

13 Voisin C, Sardella A, Marcucci F, Bernard A. Infant swimming in chlorinated pools and the risks of bronchiolitis, asthma and allergy. Eur Respir J. 2010 Jul; 36(1):41-7. doi: 10.1183/09031936.00118009. Epub 2010 Jan 14. PubMed PMID: 20075053.

RESPIRATORY

- Coughing (without fever) that does not seem to improve with time
- Congestion (without fever) that does not seem to improve with time
- Blocked nose (without fever) that does not seem to improve with time
- Runny nose (without fever) that does not seem to improve with time
- Cold-like symptoms (without fever) that does not seem to improve with time
- Difficulty breathing (any time of the day or night)
- Face goes blue
- Constant or reoccurring infections
- Wheezing
- Gasping for air

GENERAL

- Sneezing frequently
- Eczema
- Spots or rashes
- Dark marks under eyes
- Hives
- General restlessness
- Muscle pain in arms and/or legs

BEHAVIOURAL

- Sudden behavioural or mood swings
- Behavioural extremes
- Out of character behaviour not associated with illness or trauma
- Irritability not associated with tiredness

- Temper tantrums
- Excessive whining
- Excessive screaming
- Excessive clinginess
- Hyperactivity
- Aggression
  - Biting
  - Hitting
  - Spitting
  - Pinching
  - Punching
  - Kicking
- Repetition of speech
- Non-stop, senseless talk
- Food cravings
- Reluctance to smile
- Excessive fatigue
- Depression
- Refusal to stay dressed
- Refusal to be touched
- Desire to hide in darkness
- Appearing to not feel pain
- ADHD
- Hyperactivity
- Convulsions

Again, many of the symptoms in the above list can be indicative of poor sleep and tiredness, physical exhaustion, illness, or deemed as "normal" behaviour for that child. I tend to disregard the idea of "bad behaviour" in a young child as normal.

I have experienced this with my own children. For example, too much fruit juice or having fruit juice without something to slow the absorption of the sugars resulted in a massive sugar spike and the subsequent low had a drastic impact on behaviour. This is not an allergic response, but being able to spot triggers and identify impacts. As a result, I have not stopped my children from having any juice, but I choose wisely, dilute it, and give them small quantities with a meal, rather than as part of a snack.

I recommend that you become a keen observer in the life of your child and stop assuming that every "cold" is a cold. Question the status quo. If you believe your baby is suffering unduly, then ask more questions. Do not be put off by stock answers. You are the expert in your child, remember, and you should *trust* your gut instinct. Keep a food and symptom diary so that you will be able to answer the questions and demonstrate links when it comes to supporting your baby.

4 MANAGING REFLUX, SILENT REFLUX AND COLIC

4.1 WHEN REFLUX IS A PROBLEM

Reflux becomes an issue when the acid of the stomach causes pain and discomfort in the oesophagus itself. This is called GORD, gastro-oesophageal reflux disease.

It is important to listen and observe your baby's cries, behaviour and movement. If you think your baby is in pain or discomfort, chances are you are right. Trust yourself.

Signs that reflux is causing discomfort include:

- Inconsolable crying
- Screaming
- Squirming and grunting
- Painful wind or gas
- Back-arching
- Difficulty in settling
- Dislike of lying down or having nappy changed
- Inability to stay asleep for long periods of time
- Constantly unhappy baby
- Thrashing head about

None of these actions will resolve the problem. Often these babies are particularly happy when feeding, and will immediately settle down if offered milk.

Of great importance when reading the situation is determining whether symptoms are constant, such that you would not describe your baby as a "happy baby".

Displaying these symptoms does not necessarily mean that your baby needs medication for reflux. Far from it, in my view. It is the very purpose of this book to understand the *underlying cause* of the reflux, because reflux is a symptom of a primary problem, not the problem itself. In other words, treating the reflux may not treat the cause, which can continue to irritate other parts of the body even with medication.

NOTE: For the remainder of this book, the term 'reflux' is used in reference to GORD, when causing pain or discomfort for baby and problematic. This definition includes silent reflux.

4.1.1   Indications of Reflux and Silent Reflux

The list of symptoms that can indicate reflux is almost endless, so it is vitally important to be observant of your baby and watch out for what and when they are behaving in a certain manner. Since baby cannot speak, remember to observe their cries and (albeit uncoordinated) movements to tell what is going on.

If you do an online search for symptoms of reflux, you will get thousands of results of webpages listing hundreds of symptoms. Almost everything on the list I provided around allergies and intolerances is often put down to reflux.

I look at it differently. When I first made the mind-shift from looking at reflux as the problem to considering it a symptom, it was a turning point for Sunflower's unsettledness. It drove me to learn, research, read and do everything I could to educate myself about the infant digestive system and the impact that food and the environment can have on babies' delicate bodies.

Don't get me wrong. There **are** times when there is an overproduction of stomach acid, but this is rare. Your baby's stomach produces acid in response to the release of a hormone. This hormone gets released when baby is eating. Food type controls the amount of hormone released, which in turn affects the amount of stomach acid produced.

This table summarises the symptoms we often observe in "reflux babies". I explain my understanding of the symptom, and why I consider it to present as such.

	SYMPTOM	EXPLANATION
FEEDING	Frequent feeds (more than 8 times per day after the first 4 weeks)	The action of feeding soothes the oesophagus. If there is acid regurgitation from the stomach, feeding will wash the acid back down and temporarily stop it hurting. Additionally, breastmilk is a natural analgesic, so helps to relieve pain[14].
	Falling asleep during a feed	An unsettled baby is often a tried baby, and the calm and comfort that comes with feeding will help baby settle.
	Often refusing to feed	Baby can go the other way and come to associate feeding with pain. This can be from a positional aspect (they don't want to recline) or discomfort during feeding if their oesophagus is raw and painful.
	Posseting (bringing up milk then swallowing it again)	Posseting is simply regurgitation. If your baby is not in any other pain, is happy and gaining weight, posseting is nothing to worry about. It is normal. Silent-refluxers don't posset much or at all.
	Spluttering, coughing, gagging or choking during a feed	All these symptoms can result from too much air in baby's mouth when trying to drink, which is indicative of a latch issue.
		Regurgitation while feeding is a signal that something more serious is going on and should be addressed immediately by a GI specialist. This is because the act of swallowing stimulates peristaltic motion, which pushes food downwards through the entire digestive tract from mouth to bottom.
		This is why we often observe that babies have a bowel movement when they are feeding!
AFTER FEEDING	Frequent vomiting, can be projectile	As a normal part of digestion, the stomach contracts strongly after a meal. This strong contraction is designed to move food down the digestive system into the small intestine. When the LOS valve is weak, some of the stomach contents may be regurgitated. The force of the

---

14 Gray L, Miller LW, Philipp BL, Blass EM. Breastfeeding is analgesic in healthy newborns. Pediatrics. 2002 Apr;109(4):590-3. PubMed PMID: 11927701

SYMPTOM	EXPLANATION
	stomach contraction can result in projectile vomit.
Bringing up food after several hours	Milk can remain in the stomach up to 5 hours after consumption. As the strong contractions continue at intervals, they can cause food to be brought up hours later.
Gagging or choking	Food being regurgitated into the oesophagus can reach the back of the mouth where it can stimulate baby's gagging reflex. Regurgitated food can even go down the windpipe resulting in choking.
Swallowing or gulping after a feed or burp	If baby is regurgitating, there may be something in the back of the mouth that baby swallows or gulps. This can sometimes be seen with silent reflux.
Spit coming back out through nose	Baby doesn't have a strong controlled swallow mechanism in early life, and so spit or regurgitated stomach contents can enter the nasal passages and come out the nose.
Constant frequent night waking	Baby wakes in discomfort from digestive system. Lying down can make the reflux worse as stomach contents can leak back through the LOS without gravity helping food move down through the digestive system.
	Painful bloating and trapped wind in the lower abdomen can also cause baby to wake as it tries to pass causing discomfort.
Stopping breathing and sleep apnoea	If regurgitated food comes back up and gets into the oesophagus, it can then block the windpipe resulting in baby being unable to breathe.
	Sleep apnoea is associated with reflux because the tonsils and adenoids may get irritated and swollen from acid. I believe they can also become irritated and enlarged through a food intolerance, which can restrict and block the airway during sleep when the muscles around the airway relax.

SLEEP

SYMPTOM	EXPLANATION
Mostly sleeping in someone's arms or on shoulder	Babies with reflux are comfortable upright and will often be most comfortable on someone's shoulder to sleep.
Difficulty getting to sleep or needing motion to sleep (car, bouncing, buggy)	A reflux baby is often an overtired baby. As a result, the level of adrenaline in their body is forcing them to stay awake. They have been put into "fight or flight" mode, ready to do something, so they appear awake, and need external help to soothe and sleep.
Waking soon after being put down, difficulty staying asleep or restless sleep	This often depends on when baby was fed before sleep. A reflux baby, especially those with a particularly weak LOS, can experience "leakage" of stomach contents that can irritate an inflamed, "raw" or even normal oesophagus causing pain. This pain is enough to cause baby to wake. Abdominal pain can also cause so much discomfort that baby wakes.
Difficulty breathing (any time of the day or night), wheezing or coughing	With the irritation that can happen as a result of stomach acid coming back up the oesophagus, the back of the throat can become inflamed and sore, and/or the tonsils and adenoids can be enlarged, which in turn restrict the windpipe causing wheezing/breathing difficulties. As a natural response, the body will cough to try to clear mucus produced in response to the irritation from the throat.

RESPIRATORY

SYMPTOM	EXPLANATION
DIGESTIVE	
Acidic or smelly breath	The nature of the regurgitated acid is sour-tasting and smelly.
Frequent hiccoughs	Hiccoughing can be seen frequently in reflux babies who have drunk too much air. It is a natural mechanism for expelling air[15] and should be allowed to continue unless causing visible discomfort.
Tummy that is rumbly, rock hard, tender, or swollen. Abdominal pain, lots of wind, painful wind or gas, trapped wind	These symptoms can be seen in babies with reflux because: their digestive system is not able to cope with that food; or the food is not sufficiently broken down before reaching the intestines, causing it to ferment resulting in gas and air in the belly; or they swallow too much air when feeding or crying and this passes into the intestines, instead of being released upwards.
Constipation	Generally speaking, if your baby is constipated, they are not getting enough fluids. Medication and anti-reflux milks can cause constipation as they actively remove fluid from your baby's body. When constipation occurs, you must be wary of dehydration. I do not see this as an indication of reflux, but as something incorrect in baby's diet.
Diarrhoea	Diarrhoea can occur in response to a food that your baby has consumed. Baby's digestive system is often much more sensitive to foods after a bout of diarrhoea as it can literally clean out the bacteria (good and bad) from the gut.
Mucus in poo, blood in poo, green poo, black poo (except after eating a banana)	Mucus can be produced by the gut in response to an irritant or allergen. This is often observed in babies with milk allergies. If you ever find blood in your baby's poo, contact your GP immediately.
WEIGHT	
Poor weight gain, weight loss, failure to thrive	If a reflux baby is vomiting most of what they consume, not getting the calories they need, or not able to keep sufficient volumes of food in

15 Howes, D. (2012). Hiccups: A new explanation for the mysterious reflex. Bioessays, 34(6), 451–453. https://www.ncbi.nlm.nih.gov/pmc/articles/PMC3504071/

SYMPTOM	EXPLANATION

COMMUNICATION

	the body, they can lose weight. If baby vomits huge amounts constantly and is not having bowel movements, contact your GP immediately and ask about pyloric stenosis (where the lower valve out of the stomach is too tight)
Normal or excessive weight gain, large weight fluctuations	Feeding eases the discomfort of reflux, and so reflux babies can be known to comfort-eat, which can result in weight gain. If your GP tells you your baby is gaining weight and so cannot have reflux, this is not true.
Constant crying, excessive crying, high-pitched crying, painful crying, screaming, unsettled or unhappy baby, irritability	Reflux babies are suffering, uncomfortable or in pain a lot of the time. Crying is their strongest method of communication, so constant crying is a very common symptom of reflux. If baby is crying excessively, screaming in pain, then there is something wrong. Babies do not cry for no reason.

POSITIONAL

Disliking lying down, disliking having nappy changed	Gravity is a reflux baby's best friend, so anything that doesn't support gravity pulling stomach acid down through the stomach may make the refluxing action "easier" and baby unhappier as a result.
Arching back, stretching neck, thrashing about	By stretching their neck, or arching their back, baby is trying to lengthen their oesophagus, to move away from the pain and its location. Thrashing about can be baby trying to "shake off" the pain.

POSITIONAL

Drawing legs up to tummy, squirming	Painful and excessive wind is often relieved by legs drawn up to the tummy tightly. There is a reason that this position is called "wind-relieving pose" in yoga.
Sandifer's Syndrome – twitching, grimacing, arching, stiffening, and seizure-like symptoms	Sandifer's Syndrome is little-understood in its cause, but research suggests that the movements are learned behaviours used by children to reduce reflux. Kinsbourne and Oxon indicated that the "child, having hit upon this movement by chance, may have found that it temporarily

	SYMPTOM	EXPLANATION
		relieved the discomfort and therefore continued to practice the relevant movements."[16]
GENERAL	Clingy, wanting to be in arms, needing to be close to mum all the time	A reflux baby wants reassurance and comfort. The first and most basic instinctive source of this comfort is mummy.
	Lethargy, general restlessness	At quiet times, a reflux baby can display lethargy or restlessness, not being able to rest because of ongoing discomfort. Alternatively, being overtired to the point of exhaustion leaves baby with zero energy for anything else.
	Hoarse raspy voice	Refluxed stomach acid can irritate the vocal cords so baby can sound raspy or hoarse.

4.2   CAUSE OR EFFECT?

There are three common causes of infant reflux, although reflux is not strictly limited to only these:

1. Too much air in the stomach, which during digestion is forcefully removed. If it goes upwards, it brings acid with it. If it moves downwards, it causes bloating and abdominal pain and gas.
2. A food substance that baby is not yet ready to digest properly. This more often shows as abdominal pain, bloating and wind.
3. Physical issues with the stomach and GI tract.

Many of the symptoms widely listed are often attributed to reflux. In truth, the symptoms come from other sources such as tongue-tie, poor latch, food intolerances and allergies. In turn, the reflux is caused by one of these.

---

16 Kinsbourne M. Hiatus hernia with contortions of the neck. Lancet. 1964 May 16;1(7342):1058-61. PubMed PMID: 14132602.

For example, a tongue-tie can easily cause reflux due to excessive air being swallowed during a feed. In this case, baby might have many reflux symptoms, including projectile vomiting, acidic breath, painful screaming, back-arching, bloating and trapped wind; these may be diagnosed and treated as though reflux is the only problem going on. In truth, no medication will get rid of all these symptoms because the cause has not been treated. While reflux might be present as a collection of symptoms, treating the symptom and not the cause (the tongue-tie) means some symptoms might improve or disappear, but the problem persists, perhaps now invisibly, and perhaps causing further issues without us knowing.

In my 2017 survey, 60.7% of babies on medications for reflux still had ongoing symptoms. This suggests to me that medication is not tackling the root cause of the issue.

4.2.1   INGESTED AIR

Drinking or swallowing too much air can cause reflux, where a build-up of air in the stomach leads to localised pain and discomfort in the tummy. This air comes under pressure by the natural churning of the stomach and can be expelled with force causing vomiting, posseting, and irritation from acid when the stomach contents reflux into the oesophagus. Ingested air that passes through the stomach can cause bloating, abdominal distension and pain, and wind. If the air pockets are large, they can be difficult to pass and feel "stuck". Massage can help move this wind along.

Discomfort in any of these regions can result in baby being unhappy and making sure you know about it. Baby may squirm and move around to try to pass the air out. Baby may also want to be held in your arms, knowing it is safe there, regardless of what else is going on.

There are many ways that a baby can ingest air, including crying, breastfeeding or bottle-feeding.

INGESTED AIR FROM CRYING

Crying leads baby to swallow air and inconsolable crying means greater amounts of air are swallowed, because baby tends to gulp when crying this way. The more baby cries, the more air they drink and the greater discomfort they could be experiencing. It's an ongoing cycle. So the best thing to do? Break that cycle.

Babies cry for so many reasons, but if left unfixed, crying can become inconsolable and painful. I have heard of cases where baby was diagnosed with reflux, solely on the symptoms, but the actual issue was overtiredness. True story.

We *must* make the simple changes first and understand those reasons for baby showing symptoms. It's not easy. However, if it's necessary to carry your baby for a few days to ensure proper sleep and plenty of rest, then that's what it takes. If baby is unhappy being down and lets you know about it, "reflux" symptoms will worsen when baby cries inconsolably, simply because there will be more air aggravating your little one's tummy.

INGESTED AIR FROM EATING & DRINKING

When older babies start to eat, they may end up swallowing air with their food. This is where teaching baby to eat with good technique is important. This means trying to show mouth closed, not talking and chatting when eating. Mindful eating is valuable to demonstrate to baby, especially if you are witnessing a "reflux flare-up" with the introduction of solids.

Additionally, if baby is using a straw to drink, they will be drinking air because the first part of the straw is filled with air. If you want to teach your baby to drink without air, use vessels like the 360° sippy cup.

INGESTED AIR FROM STRUCTURAL ISSUES

All babies go through trauma during birth, regardless of birthing method. However, it is more likely that if there is any intervention during birth, that the natural movement of the spinal column and cranial bones may not complete fully, and that residual misalignments, tension and stresses remain in baby's body. If these misalignments are high in the spine, in the head and / or jaw bones, they can have a very immediate and direct impact on baby's ability to have full free motion of their head and mouth for feeding effectively. Ineffective feeding can result in air being swallowed, and this can result in reflux and colic.

Western medicine does not typically deal with these micro mis-alignments because they are not obvious. However, there are two specific therapists who are qualified to assess the structural alignment of the body and make micro adjustments to resolve tension: paediatric chiropractic and cranio-sacral osteopathy.

Indications that your baby may require support with the alignment of their body include (and are not limited to) the following:

- Intervention during birth
  - Induction
  - Assisted delivery
    - Forceps
    - Suction cup / Ventouse
    - Help from midwife / obstetrician during delivery (e.g. twisting, pulling, anything other than free birth)
  - C-section (emergency or planned)
  - Epidural
  - Mother being in laid back position during birth
  - Delayed labour
- Position of baby after birth
  - Baby appears to feed more comfortably on one side than the other
  - Baby sleeps with head extended
  - Plagiocephaly (flat head)
  - Torticollis (twisted neck, tilted head position)

INGESTED AIR IN FROM TONGUE-TIE

Too much air may also be swallowed because of a tongue-tie (ankyloglossia), regardless of how baby is fed. There is a myth that tongue-tie is only important in breastfed babies. This simply is not true. The movement of the tongue is massively important in both breast- and bottle-fed infants, as they need to use their tongue to reduce the volume of air in their mouth.

An International Board Certified Lactation Consultant, or a Tongue-Tie practitioner can assess your baby's latch and advise if a tongue-tie is present, and advise who can resolve it. In a baby who is swallowing too much air, there is no such thing as a tongue-tie that is not affecting how they feed, it should be resolved.

Tongue-tie also has a much greater impact than just feeding. See section 4.3 Tongue-Tie & Reflux (page 60) for more information.

Bottle-fed infants are also susceptible to drinking too much air, particularly as bottle teats do not deform the way a nipple does. Added to that, most bottles have a natural flow, which means baby does not have to suck; the action which naturally removes excess air from their mouth before swallowing.

If you see your baby spilling or leaking milk from the mouth while feeding, there is too much air being drunk. If milk can get out, air can get in. Add a tongue-tie into the mix and this makes bottle-feeding even more difficult. A bottle-fed baby with a tongue-tie will rarely feed easily or happily. Babies should be assessed for a tongue-tie if you're experiencing this difficulty. I recommend you find a tongue-tie practitioner to assess and resolve. (http://www.tongue-tie.org.uk/)

WINDING

If you have identified that your baby is consuming too much air, go to town on moving the air up and out of the stomach before it passes down and causes abdominal discomfort. The more wind and air you can release from baby's tummy as possible during and after feeding. There are many techniques and methods for releasing wind, and a quick search on YouTube will show you many that you may not be aware of already. Additionally, my e-courses have additional and constantly updated information on supporting your baby with various techniques by other professionals.

4.2.2   FOOD REACTIONS

If all latch issues have been ruled out, it may be that baby has an intolerance or allergy to the milk they are drinking. Breastfed infants cannot have an allergy to the breastmilk itself, but rather a substance in the breastmilk which is present because of mum's diet and/or environment. (See Section 4.4 Breastfeeding & Reflux page 63 for more details). On the plus side, mum has total control over what goes into her milk, because she sets her own diet and environment. Removing major allergens from a mother's diet can have a massive impact on baby's "reflux". The major allergens in question are dairy and beef, gluten, eggs and nuts. I explain this in greater detail in Section **Error! Reference source not found. Error! Reference source not found.** page **Error! Bookmark not defined.**).

Cow's milk protein allergy, or CMPA, presents with the same symptoms as reflux, and is often treated with reflux medication first. When the treatment does not work, a change in milk is normally advised and mum is told to switch to a non-dairy milk. Personally, I feel potential changes in milk should be trialled before strong reflux medications; it is easier for baby's body without having to cope with strong medications that are generally not proven safe in infants under 12 months old by the manufacturers.

By keeping a food and symptom diary, you can track down which foods could be causing symptoms.

If your breastfed baby has reflux or CMPA, the best way to minimise impact by milk on your baby's immature digestive system is to keep breastfeeding and change what you eat. A change in diet, coupled with a latch assessment, tongue-tie rectification (if needed) and breastfeeding support, can provide your baby with a new lease of life. In some cases, there may be some issues not dealt with by milk alone, and these cases are where medication may be needed to get your baby to a place of complete happiness.

For bottle-fed babies, specialist milks are available. Due to the differing ingredients across brands, no one milk is any better than another for babies in general. To find out what is right for *your* child, it's simply a matter of trial and error. I have detailed more about some of the major formula brands in Section 6.1 Formula Milks page 125).

Lastly, baby could be ingesting foods that are fermenting in their gut because of their naturally immature digestion capability, causing abdominal pain and distention, or allergens that are causing other reactions like skin conditions such as eczema and hives. All signs from baby and baby's body are clues to put together and figure out what is going on for your little one.

Once you discover the real root of the problem, "reflux" is much easier to fix.

4.2.3   PHYSICAL ISSUES

What I've mentioned so far is not the extent of all the problems out there. There may be something more serious going on that has not been picked up. In rare cases, babies present with reflux but actually have a more dangerous condition going on, such as necrotising enterocolitis, pyloric stenosis, a blockage in the intestine or a motility issue in which the peristaltic action of the digestive system does not function correctly. There may be many more examples of physical issues where reflux results. I advocate a "better safe than sorry" mandate, so advise you to seek medical advice if you suspect these conditions for your baby.

Remember these are incredibly rare and must be identified early to help baby as quickly as possible. For further information, read Section 4.10 Associated Conditions & Symptoms (page 99).

4.3   TONGUE-TIE & REFLUX

Note: For All babies with feeding discomfort, please check out the updated Oral Play and Tongue Tie online course which explores oral function in much greater detail than is available in this book. www.thebabyrefluxlady.co.uk/book-reader

This is a bit of a hobby horse of mine. Through my private work, I've found many babies with a tongue-tie. They have been assessed by their GP, health visitor or breastfeeding counsellor and been given the all clear, or told that baby does have a tongue-tie but it is not affecting their feeding so they do not need to do anything about it. False.

Firstly, I respect the work that GPs, health visitors and breastfeeding counsellors do, but they are not qualified to diagnose a tongue-tie. Some tongue-ties are so severe that anyone could see it. (For example, mine! Visit my Facebook page to see it!) Yet there are tongue-ties that are virtually impossible to see with your eye, and need very specific skills to diagnose. These tongue-ties can have a very real and direct impact on baby's drinking ability and reflux.

I choose to not believe anyone who says that there is a tongue-tie present but it is not affecting baby enough to have it resolved.

Absolutely false.

Further to this, I see mums agonising over the decision of whether or not to have a tongue-tie cut, especially when baby is a little older, 5 months, 11 months, or more. I always advise to have it cut. A tongue-tie does not just impact feeding and reflux.

There are longer-term developmental and digestive impacts to not having proper tongue freedom. If the tongue cannot move freely in the mouth, it will be difficult to adequately mix food with saliva before swallowing, limiting the exposure of food to salivary amylase, an extremely important part of digestion in babies up until 2 to 2½ years of age.

If the tongue cannot move properly, baby may find it difficult to make proper shapes in their mouth for speech development, causing delayed communication, speech and language difficulties.

If the tongue is tied to the floor of the mouth it cannot push against the teeth properly and results in a narrow jaw development presenting as overcrowded teeth. The tongue is also responsible for the development of the upper palate. With proper tongue movement, the upper palate of the mouth drags downwards and widens out. Without this, the child may grow up to have a narrow palate and require extensive orthodontic treatment[17].

17http://www.drghaheri.com/blog/2016/6/23/breastfeeding-compensations-for-tonguelip-tie-are-problematic

So you see how a tongue-tie can cause reflux, and is highly important. Even if medication addresses the reflux symptoms, there are longer-term gains to having the tongue-tie resolved. In an infant, it takes less than a minute and offers a lifetime of benefits.

And then there is the aftercare that goes with having a tongue-tie cut. There are schools of thought that no aftercare is needed and others go so far as encouraging you to physically break through any scar tissue that has formed overnight each morning.

Having been through both, I found my way. I do not believe in zero aftercare. For the most up-to-date information on pre and post care for all babies with feeding challenges, *please check out the Oral Play and Tongue Tie online* www.thebabyrefluxlady.co.uk/book-reader

Breaking it down into what happens... If a tongue-tie has been released, baby has suddenly got a massive amount of new found freedom of movement. Baby uses this freedom of movement, and guess what? It hurts. But not because it was cut.

What happens when you exercise a muscle in a way you haven't done before, or for a long time? Yes – it hurts after a few days. Sometimes it hurts so much you can barely move at all.

The tongue is a muscle. Could baby be suffering with pain in their tongue a few days after a tongue-tie release? Seems plausible enough to me.

When Daffodil's tongue was released the second time, and it pained me so much to witness it, I was given a very strict and intrusive aftercare regime to follow. I tried. I tried so hard, because I wanted her to not have reflux anymore and I'd had a glimpse of what she could be like without it when her tongue had been released the first time. I did it with pain in my heart the first morning after. It was such a harrowing experience that I couldn't bring myself to do it again.

The aftercare exercises we were given were to be done every 2 hours or so during the day, and first thing in the morning (when I would have to 'break' the scar tissue). Instead, I decided to figure out what the aftercare was doing for her. I realised that what she needed to do was to keep moving her tongue, move it enough such that the wound did not sit on itself long enough to start forming scar tissue again.

So I figured out that no matter what was going on, Daffodil would have milk. Her happiest place was on boob. And given that this was also the most effective place for her to extend her "new" tongue, while providing an analgesic effect, this was going to be the basis of my own aftercare.

For 3 days and nights, I fed her every 2 hours. Not for long, but long enough so that I was confident her tongue was moving properly. I concentrated on getting her latch perfect, encouraging her to open her mouth wider than before and supporting her. I set my alarm to wake us both during the night.

I accepted that feeding every 2 hours was not practical, but 3 days of this was not going to be long enough to become a new routine. After 3 days of feeding every 2 hours around the clock, I shifted it to every 3 hours for another 4 days and nights. After a week, I was confident that the wound was not going to stick to itself again. (I also did some finger games with her tongue to make sure I could see under it.) At that point, I let us slip back into a more natural rhythm. This was our solution, and it worked for us.

I encourage every parent who is getting a tongue-tie released to have a full understanding of what you need to look out for and how to care for it in the days and weeks after, as well as what to do if you think it is sticking. Regardless of how you feed your baby, get their tongue-tie assessed and resolved as early as possible. Then be gentle with them. And remember, they must *learn* how to use their new tongue.

4.4   BREASTFEEDING & REFLUX

It is shocking that breastfeeding mums are so often told to stop breastfeeding as a first step, when reflux is suspected, and switch to formula milk. There is nothing wrong with your breastmilk!

Breastmilk is your baby's *perfect food*. It is designed *by nature* to be the perfect food. It is the greatest known superfood on earth. It has the capacity to nourish your child like nothing else, because your child is unique and so is your breastmilk.

Your body responds to your baby through almost magical interactions[18] and feedback mechanisms during feeding to provide the best balance of nutrients and minerals they need from day to day.

Breastmilk as a substance *does not cause* reflux. There is also no such thing as an allergy to breastmilk. There is galactosaemia, when a newborn cannot tolerate *any* milk. This is not an allergy. It is an inability of baby's liver to digest galactose in the milk. This is an extremely serious life-threatening condition and newborns with this disorder need an extremely high level of care in the first few days of life, including a specialised feeding regime to survive.

Incredibly rare, galactosaemia affects between 1 in 16,000 and 1 in 48,000 infants. A survey I conducted in 2017 found that mothers were being told their baby could be allergic to their breastmilk at a rate 2,500 times greater than the true occurrence of this devastating condition. This represents a gross misunderstanding of the truth about breastmilk and its composition.

Every substance in a breastfeeding mother's circulation has the potential to get into the infant's body and should be considered a potential irritant, independent to the breastmilk itself. Thankfully, you can remove irritants from your diet and environment, which I've found, both personally and with clients in my private practice, can resolve many reflux-related issues.

In fact, if baby is breastfed and showing signs of reflux, breastmilk is the best source of food, not least because it is the easiest to influence. You

---

18 Donna T. Ramsay, Jacqueline C. Kent, Robyn A. Owens, Peter E. Hartmann, Ultrasound Imaging of Milk Ejection in the Breast of Lactating Women, Pediatrics, February 2004, VOLUME 113 / ISSUE 2

can do a lot to minimise the air a baby drinks when breastfeeding, you can do so much to resolve tongue-tie and you can do massive amounts with diet modification to minimise the impact breastmilk has on reflux symptoms.

There are several other reasons why breastmilk is helpful when it comes to reflux. Firstly, it contains a natural analgesic, so it's essentially a painkiller for baby! Secondly, the act of suckling and feeding stimulates peristalsis and makes everything move in the correct downward direction. And thirdly, milk will wash back down any acid that is annoying baby. Finally, while your breastmilk may have particles in it that your baby cannot digest properly, you can change this situation with relative ease. Formula milk is formula milk; you cannot change what is in it. There are few formulas (if any) that are properly digestible by infants, so many parents try various types of milk with worsening symptoms. Even more amazing, in 7.4% of reflux babies, reflux only started after breastfeeding was stopped.

4.5   Tummy Action & Reflux

You may observe a pattern whereby the reflux-related behaviours and upper respiratory tract irritation are at their worst 30 or 90 minutes after a feed. This is because the stomach, as part of the digestive process, makes two strong contractions, designed to move food out of the stomach, usually down into the small intestine, approximately 30 minutes and again 90 minutes after eating.

This happens in everyone, but in babies with reflux, this is when acid and food come back out of the stomach upwards. Unlike the intestine, the oesophagus does not have a buffer to protect it from stomach acid, hence your baby's pain or discomfort.

If you notice a distinct pattern like this, you can put in place a strategy that maximises your baby's chance of rest. For example, keeping them upright for 30 minutes after a feed, and then putting them down for a nap to get a hour's rest until the next stomach contraction, which may or may not wake them.

4.6   MISSED & MISDIAGNOSIS OF REFLUX

In my opinion, there appears to be gross missed diagnoses and misdiagnoses of reflux. With **67%** of respondents to my reflux survey saying they did not receive adequate support from their primary carer (GP, health visitor, midwife, paediatrician) for their baby's reflux. I have *hundreds* of stories from real mums, of real babies, who believe they have been ignored, have had to fight for their babies, have been told "baby has colic", have experienced no official diagnosis from their healthcare providers and have used the internet to get a diagnosis (like me), or felt like they were alone in this.

This is a massive problem for parents and babies. Consultants and GPs seem all too happy to prescribe medications for young infants with complete disregard for long-term consequences, necessity or effectiveness. Perhaps they feel pressured into it by relentless mums who *demand* particular medications for their babies; but this *only* happens because the parents feel that they are not listened to in the first place.

When medications do not work, the apparent norm is to try another medication and another. I know many babies who are on multiple drugs, still with no effect or improvement in symptoms.

The table overleaf shows the proportion of babies who continue to suffer with reflux-type symptoms, and which medications, if any they are taking. The most striking thing is that 88.6% of babies who still suffer with reflux symptoms are on prescription medication. 76.3% are on acid-blocking medication, for which a known side effect is "gastrointestinal disturbances".

Is our approach to blanket medication become iatrogenic? Are the medications causing more problems than they are solving?

Clearly, the medications are not 100% effective most of the time, so there **must** be something else going on.

Of the Children Still Experiencing Reflux Symtpoms, which (if any) medications are they taking?

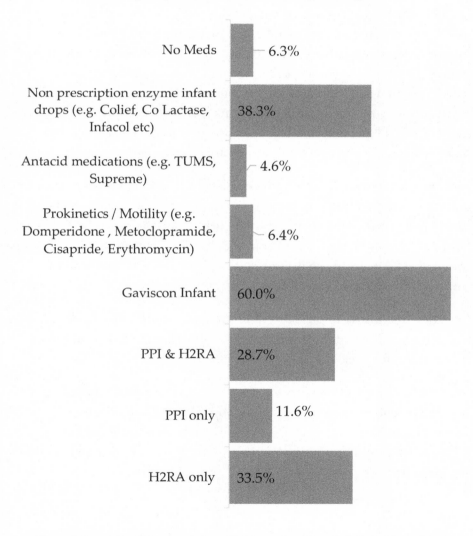

Figure 2 shows that of the population of babies and toddlers (1,499), 61.4% continue to suffer with reflux symptoms (920), and 73.8% of this population are still taking acid-blocking

medications, for which gastrointestinal disturbances are listed as side effects.
Source: Reflux Survey carried out by Aine Homer, May 2017 – July 2018

Surely, the question we should be asking here is: *what is the root cause?* Surely, we should stop thinking along the lines of: *what other medication can we try?* Medicine in the West seems so far removed from what healthcare should be. It is all about managing symptoms, rather than understanding why they are present and tackling that.

In my survey of parents of babies with reflux, when asked about misdiagnoses, there were several cases, including a child having been diagnosed as a reflux baby who turned out to be overtired. In my own family, Daffodil was prescribed strong anti-reflux medication by our paediatrician when the cause was a tongue-tie. I was told, "She does not have a tongue-tie; she has reflux". Thankfully, I stuck to my own guns. I never filled the prescription but went privately to have her tongue-tie resolved and *this* changed her life and mine.

One of the most common missed diagnoses is food intolerances, in particular cow's milk protein allergy. CMPA can be severe, to the point that a baby could have an anaphylactic reaction. Baby might be displaying "reflux" symptoms, but is intolerant or allergic to something in milk. Most often, CMPA tends to be diagnosed after baby does not respond to prescription medication for reflux.

The same theory applies to solid food and baby, a breastfeeding mother can alter her diet and digestion (for example, through improved mastication for breakdown of starches).

By following a simple diet for a few days, a breastfeeding mother can massively reduce symptoms in their baby. Then, through careful reintroduction of foods, she may identify those that upset her baby's digestive system. Using a food and symptom diary is a great asset in this endeavour.

4.7   The Basics of Helping Baby

If your baby is having symptoms associated with food and/or air coming up from the stomach, regurgitation of any sort, there are a few simple techniques you can try to support their body.

Remember, gravity has a big part to play, with your baby benefitting simply from being more upright for longer after a feed.

- Use gravity to your baby's advantage
  - o Sit baby in a more upright position while feeding
  - o Hold baby upright for longer after a feed (for example, in a carrier)
  - o Raise the head of their bed by about 4 inches using books or blocks of wood under the crib feet
  - o Get a quality carrier (see my website for personal recommendations). Baby will be comforted just by being close to you, reducing the amount of air they swallow when crying. They can happily nap in there while you get on with stuff.
  - o Get a good quality swing that will rock them for day-time naps.
  - o Change nappies before a feed to avoid changing it immediately after.
- Co-sleep safely if you're comfortable with it. The night-time closeness of mum can be magical.
- Reduce the size of each feed.
- For bottles, stir to mix, don't shake. Shaking introduces air into the milk itself.
- Wind for longer during and after each feed. Use YouTube to find new techniques you may not have tried.
- Try changing to the Medela Calma bottle and teat (http://geni.us/Medela).
- Try adding infant digestive enzymes such as Colief to milk. (Not for dairy-intolerant babies as the lactase is derived from cow's milk.)

- Loosen nappy to avoid too much pressure on abdomen. Avoid clothes like jeans that are tight around the belly. Opt for leggings, dresses, tracksuits, or even better, sleepsuits.
- White noise can help soothe sometimes.
- Sing! Mum's voice is so comforting to little ones that recording yourself singing a lullaby and playing it back can help baby to settle.
- Wear a cardigan or top for a few hours, then put it beside baby when sleeping, or in another person's arms so that they can smell you.
- Try infant massage. Watch examples on YouTube and find a local class to attend.

It is unlikely that any single one of these suggestions will rid your baby of their symptoms completely, they may make life much more comfortable.

4.8   NON-MEDICAL SOLUTIONS FOR REFLUX

There are several complementary therapies that can support your infant through any reflux issues they may be experiencing. Each therapy offers something different so it is important to find out what you think supports your baby best. If you can understand the cause of the reflux or colic first, then you will be able to find a helpful therapy more easily, as you will know where to look for a specific resolution.

This list is not exhaustive, and there are many other therapies out there. Do your research and find out what might work for your baby. Understand your baby's cause of discomfort and what the therapy proposes to do. If the therapy sounds like it may help, then try. If not, do not be afraid to thank the therapist for their time and leave it to the side.

You are making decisions on behalf of your baby. I *know* the exhaustion and the desperation to help your baby are your driver, so channel these into making the best decision.

Do not be taken in by trying everything. Not everything will work. Every case of reflux is different and there are different solutions for every baby.

For all complementary therapies, best results are achieved with an accurate description of all the symptoms that you observe in your infant, including severity, time of day and other information. The more detail you can describe, the better the outcome, as the practitioner will be able to identify subtleties in presenting patterns and treat accordingly.

4.8.1   ACUPUNCTURE

Acupuncture is a traditional form of Eastern medicine that uses needles (or pressure in acupressure) to stimulate specific points around the body. Acupuncture rebalances the infant's system by stimulating a pattern of points.

It can be extremely powerful in supporting the infant digestive system, strengthening the LOS, rebalancing the acid amount, and reducing pain. If there is a physical cause for reflux, such as repeated drinking of too much air, acupuncture cannot resolve the problem.

Acupuncture has been successfully shown to have reduced symptoms in colicky babies[19].

4.8.2   CHIROPRACTIC

Chiropractic is the diagnosis and treatment of mechanical disorders of the musculoskeletal system, especially the spine. A chiropractor will make tiny adjustments of the infant's spine and skeleton to ensure the body is properly aligned, since misalignment can introduce stress and illness into the body.

An infant's skeletal system can easily be misaligned from the positioning in the womb and the amount of space in the last few weeks of pregnancy,

---

19 Landgren, Kajsa; Hallström, Inge; Effect of minimal acupuncture for infantile colic: a multicentre, three-armed, single-blind, randomised controlled trial (ACU-COL), June 2017 Acupunct Med 2017;35:171–179. doi:10.1136/acupmed-2016-011208

the birthing process, and from movements made when in pain, such as over-extension of their head and neck, and arching that we so often see in reflux.

4.8.3   CRANIOSACRAL THERAPY

Craniosacral therapy is gentle manipulation of the bones of the skull to ensure proper alignment. It includes the bones, membranes and fluids around the brain and spinal cord as well as the attached bones – skull, face, jaw and tailbone (sacrum).

It is easy to see how the bones of an infant's skull could be misaligned after a vaginal birth, especially with intervention such as ventouse or forceps. As with chiropractic, the general understanding is that skeletal misalignment introduces stresses into the body, which can manifest in many ways. If there is a misalignment in the skull that affects how baby is feeding, this can have a direct impact on reflux from latch issues.

4.8.4   DIETARY MODIFICATION & SUPPLEMENTS

Frequently there are substances in your baby's milk (breast or formula) that they cannot digest. In my Food for Reflux Babies coaching practice, I support mums to identify foods that are sources of irritation for their babies and to eliminate them. It is not unusual to see their babies' reflux virtually disappear within days of changing their own diet. See section 9 Foundations of Change (page 186) for more information on this for breastfed babies.

Depending on the source of your baby's reflux or colic, this solution may help or it may not. Again, understanding the cause is all-important for treating the symptoms.

COCONUT OIL

Coconut oil is famed for its antibacterial and antimicrobial properties. Empirical evidence suggests that coconut oil can support your baby's digestive system by lubricating it. Not only is the lauric acid a well-known anti-inflammatory, but the oil coats the oesophagus, protecting it from acid regurgitation and allowing it to heal.

In addition, coconut oil is the best-known source of medium chain triglycerides (MCTs), an essential fatty acid already broken down, and an amazing source of pure energy. It is absorbed without need for further digestion so if you are worried about your baby's energy intake, coconut oil can support this.

General recommendations are about 1 teaspoon per a day. I suggest splitting this amount of coconut oil across the number of feeds your baby has so that there is protective oil in each feed. You can mix the oil in with your baby's milk or swab it around their mouth.

I recommend an organic, aroma-free, cold-pressed coconut oil for your baby.

As with everything I suggest, be wary when introducing a new food substance as there is always the possibility that it may cause an adverse reaction.

PROBIOTICS

Probiotics are bacteria essential for proper digestion and function of the bowel. All the research points towards positive outcomes for use of probiotics for infantile colic. These studies are all in relation to one specific strain – *Lactobacillus reuteri* DSM 17938, a particular lactic acid bacteria.

Research from 2014 concluded that "early administration of *L. reuteri* DSM 17938 resulted beneficial in preventing regurgitation episodes during the first month of life."[20] Another paper reached the conclusion that probiotics should be used as a preventative measure: "Prophylactic use of *L. reuteri* DSM 17938 during the first 3 months of life reduced the magnitude of crying and functional gastrointestinal disorders."[21]

---

20 Garofoli F, Civardi E, Indrio F, Mazzucchelli I, Angelini M, Tinelli C, Stronati M. The early administration of Lactobacillus reuteri DSM 17938 controls regurgitation episodes in full-term breastfed infants. Int J Food Sci Nutr. 2014 Aug;65(5):646-8. doi: 10.3109/09637486.2014.898251. Epub 2014 Mar 17. PubMed PMID: 24635827.
21 Chumpitazi BP, Shulman RJ. Prophylactic use of probiotics ameliorates infantile colic. J Pediatr. 2014 Jul;165(1):210. doi: 10.1016/j.jpeds.2014.04.026. PubMed PMID: 24973164; PubMed Central PMCID: PMC4413909.

Probiotics are particularly recommended for children who have suffered with diarrhoea, which wipes out the healthy bacteria of the gut and can mark the beginning of a bout of digestive discomfort.

My recommendation are the BioGaia Protectis Drops, made from this beneficial bacterium and free from milk, though these drops do contain traces of gluten as the probiotic is cultured on barley[22]. http://geni.us/BioGaia

CAUTION: When selecting probiotics, take good care if you suspect any dairy intolerance or allergy, as most probiotics are derived from dairy sources. Read carefully and make sure you understand the ingredients. Some probiotics will say they are "suitable for lactose-intolerant people", but this does not apply if there is a protein allergy in play.

DIGESTIVE ENZYMES

Colief is a brand of digestive enzymes, specifically for the digestion and breakdown of lactose. If it is a lactose intolerance that is causing your baby's abdominal discomfort, this product may help with the digestion of milk sugars and reduce the formation of gas in the intestine.

CAUTION: If you know your child to have CMPA, do not use these drops as they are derived from milk sources.

ESSENTIAL OILS

Some essential oils are documented to have beneficial properties for the digestive system. Given the number of brands available, and variation in oil concentration and quality, I do not make any specific recommendations here, except to say do not use essential oils internally with infants and young children due to their potency.

HERBAL TEAS

There are a number of herbal teas that have been produced with baby in mind and that are therefore safe to use for infants. Neuners do a Baby Stomach Tea, which includes aniseed, fennel, camomile, caraway and

---

22 https://www.biogaia.com/product-country/biogaia-protectis-drops-33/

thyme in dilution concentrations safe and beneficial for baby. You may find that a tea such as this supports baby's digestive system in terms of passing gas, reducing bloating etc. It will not address the root cause of the problem.

GRIPE WATER

Gripe water is a blend of herbs, specifically designed for relief from stomach pains. Typically, it works by popping large air bubbles in the stomach and letting them escape by more effective winding, and by neutralising stomach acid.

Infacol is an anti-flatulent, meaning it helps to bring up wind trapped in the tummy. It is safe to use from birth. And its active ingredient is simethicone[23].

CAUTION: With the exception of Infacol, gripe waters should not be used before 1 month old.

4.8.5   HOMEOPATHY

Homeopathy is a form of natural medicine based on the doctrine "like cures like" – that a substance that causes the symptoms of a disease in healthy people would cure similar symptoms in sick people.

A consultation with a homeopath will be like a detailed interview, describing symptoms, time of day, emotions and such like.

Care with homeopathic remedy should be observed, as tissue salts and tablets are made with lactose, which may cause more upset in babies. The best options are pillules, which are made with sucrose, or tinctures that you mix with water. You must get specific guidance from a qualified homeopath for use of tinctures safely due to potency levels.

---

23 http://www.medicines.org.uk/emc/PIL.15524.latest.pdf

The correct remedy for your baby will very much depend on the specifics of their symptoms and personality, so consultation with a registered homeopath is recommended.

One liquid homeopathic remedy designed with baby colic and reflux in mind is ColicCalm. It is a remedy of nine herbs for treating a variety of symptoms[24]. Speaking from personal experience, this helped relieve wind in my daughter Daffodil, although I didn't try it with silent reflux because I didn't yet know about it.

4.8.6   OSTEOPATHY

Osteopathy is the manipulation of bones and tissues of the body to ensure alignment and removal of stresses. As with other therapies, the understanding is that misalignments in the body will introduce stress, which can manifest in multiple guises.

We forget that the birthing process is a massive physical ordeal for baby's body. They, too, go through some massive physical strains as well as mum. Baby's skull is designed to move, for the bones to overlap each other during birth. If your baby's body is not realigned with itself shortly after birth, the invisible misalignments can introduce stress and discomfort.

The ability to apply feather-light touch to influence the alignment of the body is a great skill to support our infants. In addition to physical alignment, osteopathy can treat the nervous system to reduce stressors within the body.

A cranial osteopath who has specialist training in paediatrics can adjust your baby and help their body settle into their new life. This alone can result in massive change for baby's latch, sleep and digestive system function.

Make sure your osteopath has infant experience. You can find a craniosacral osteopath (often shortened to cranio-osteopath) who has

---

24 https://www.coliccalm.co.uk/blog/baby_colic_treatment#SodiumBicarb

additional training in craniosacral therapy, giving your baby more benefits from one practitioner.

The sooner after birth you can see a craniosacral osteopath the better. Most osteopaths will treat babies from 2 weeks old. Repeat treatments may be required as baby's body goes through such rapid growth and development.

4.8.7   REFLEXOLOGY

This is the application of pressure and massage to various parts of the feet. The soles of the feet are divided into zones that correspond to other parts of the body. Massage and pressure can relieve pain and discomfort, or stimulate specific actions in the body.

I learned a simple set of massage strokes for supporting the digestive system. When I used them with Daffodil during her first few weeks of upset (before her tongue-tie was released), it helped trapped and painful wind to pass quickly and easily. Since then, it has helped with trapped wind from food.

4.8.8   INFANT MASSAGE

Infant massage is when a caregiver applies gentle strokes and massage to areas of baby's body. The massage offers bonding and communication opportunities, and has several benefits for reflux babies. Infant massage can help with the movement of wind and food through the digestive system, reduce constipation, and ease colic.

While this does not offer a cure, it can certainly help ease symptoms and support restful sleep; plus, it can give dads a meaningful intervention to bond with baby, so long as baby is comfortable lying down.

If baby has a strong dislike of lying down, you can sit them on your knee and move their upper body in a circular manner to stretch and compress the intestines. This can help air move upwards and downwards.

4.9   MEDICAL SOLUTIONS & WHERE TO FIND THEM

NICE management guidelines are a resource available to the general public as well as being the guidelines that our GPs should follow. While they do not mention discovering the *cause* in the early stages of feeding (for example, assessing tongue-tie and latch for formula-fed babies or simple understanding of the substances that may be in breastmilk or formula that are irritating baby's immature digestive system), I welcome the guidelines, because they do not condone ignoring symptoms.

NICE recommends that a GP should refer a child with GORD in the following scenarios[25]:

- "Arrange same-day admission if any of the following are present:
    o Haematemesis (not caused by swallowed blood from a nosebleed or a cracked nipple)
    o Melaena (black, foul-smelling stool)
    o Dysphagia
- Arrange a specialist assessment by a paediatrician or paediatric gastroenterologist (the urgency of referral depending on clinical judgement) if there is:
    o An uncertain diagnosis or red flag symptoms that suggest a more serious condition
    o Persistent, faltering growth associated with regurgitation
    o Unexplained distress in children with communication difficulties
    o Symptoms suggestive of GORD needing ongoing medical therapy or not responding to medical therapy
    o Feeding aversion and a history of regurgitation
    o Unexplained iron deficiency anaemia
    o No improvement in regurgitation after 1 year of age
    o Suspected Sandifer's Syndrome

---

25 https://cks.nice.org.uk/gord-in-children#!scenario

- Refer to a paediatrician or paediatric gastroenterologist if there is a suspected complication (the urgency of referral depending on clinical judgement) such as:
  o Suspected recurrent aspiration pneumonia
  o Unexplained apnoeas (periods of stopping breathing in sleep)
  o Unexplained epileptic seizure-like events
  o Unexplained upper airway inflammation
  o Dental erosion associated with a neurodisability
  o Recurrent acute otitis media (ear infections) already managed appropriately."

4.9.1   DIAGNOSTIC TOOLS

GASTROINTESTINAL CONTRAST STUDY

A GI contrast study – also known as oesophagram or barium swallow – is an x-ray of the digestive system while it is coated with barium. This type of study allows specialists to understand and see how your baby's digestive system is working. It is used to diagnose all types of abnormalities of the digestive system[26].

- Follow-through scans are used to show your child's oesophagus and stomach, but mainly the small intestine.
- Contrast meal scans and contrast swallow scans are used to study the oesophagus and stomach in detail.

Baby would usually only be referred for this if there are red flag symptoms presenting that warrant further inspection, and if your child is not responding well to other medical intervention.

Having a GI contrast study is recommended as an urgent, same-day assessment where:

---

26 http://www.gosh.nhs.uk/medical-information/procedures-and-treatments/upper-gi-contrast-study-including-barium-meal-barium-swallow-or-barium-follow-through-studies

- There is unexplained bile-stained vomiting to rule out more serious disorders such as intestinal obstruction.
- The infant is less than 2 months old and presents with worsening or forceful vomiting of feeds to assess for possible hypertrophic pyloric stenosis.

A GI contrast study should be scheduled where there is:

- History of dysphagia (difficulty swallowing); or
- Ongoing history of bile-stained vomiting.

NICE guidelines state, "Do not offer an upper gastrointestinal (GI) contrast study to diagnose or assess severity of GORD in infants, children and young people."[27]

UPPER GASTROINTESTINAL ENDOSCOPY

A gastrointestinal paediatrician or surgeon will use an endoscope to look inside an infant's upper GI tract. This is often used if there is suspicion of erosive oesophageal (EE), where the acid from the stomach has inflamed and worn away the lining of the oesophagus.

Indications for a GI endoscopy in infants with GORD are:

1. Failure to respond to prescription medication
2. Unexplained anaemia
3. Faecal occult blood
4. Recurrent pneumonia
5. Haematemesis (blood-stained vomit)
6. Malaena (black, foul-smelling stool)
7. Dysphagia (difficulty swallowing)
8. No improvement in regurgitation after 1 year old persistent
9. Faltering growth associated with overt regurgitation

27 https://www.nice.org.uk/guidance/ng1/resources/gastrooesophageal-reflux-disease-in-children-and-young-people-diagnosis-and-management-pdf-51035086789

10. Unexplained distress in children and young people with communication difficulties
11. Retrosternal (behind the sternum in the upper chest), epigastric or upper abdominal pain that needs ongoing medical therapy or is not responding to medical therapy
12. Feeding aversion and a history of regurgitation
13. Unexplained iron-deficiency anaemia
14. Suspected diagnosis of Sandifer's Syndrome

Indications 1-5 are the precursors as recommended by the North American Society of Paediatric Gastroenterology, Hepatology and Nutrition[28]. Indications 5-14 are outlined in the UK's NICE Guidelines from 2015[29].

OESOPHAGEAL pH STUDY/pH PROBE

A pH probe monitors stomach acid close to the lower oesophageal valve. A long tube with the probe at one end is required to remain in place for 24 hours.

A 2001 study outlined that "oesophageal pH monitoring cannot reliably detect GOR in pre-term infants"[30] and that it should not be used in those infants.

The UK's NICE guidelines for performing a pH study cover infants and children with:

- Suspected recurrent aspiration pneumonia
- Unexplained apnoeas
- Unexplained non-epileptic seizure-like events
- Unexplained upper airway inflammation
- Dental erosion associated with a neurodisability
- Frequent otitis media

---

28 http://www.giejournal.org/article/S0016-5107(15)00147-9/pdf
29 https://www.nice.org.uk/guidance/ng1/resources/gastrooesophageal-reflux-disease-in-children-and-young-people-diagnosis-and-management-pdf-51035086789
30 Grant L, Cochran D Can pH monitoring reliably detect gastro-oesophageal reflux in pre-term infants? Archives of Disease in Childhood – Fetal and Neonatal Edition 2001;85:F155-F158

- Possible need for surgery that wraps the upper part of the stomach around the lower end of the oesophagus to reinforce the closing function of the LOS[31] (fundoplication)
- Suspected diagnosis of Sandifer's Syndrome.

4.9.2   MEDICATION FOR REFLUX

Medication has become the standard way of treating reflux, though medication only treats the symptoms and rarely treat the root cause of the reflux. It is extremely rare for a baby to have "acid reflux". Acid reflux is a specific term given to the over-production of stomach acid.

In reflux babies, even those officially diagnosed with GORD, there is not an over-production of acid. They are extremely uncomfortable, and in pain, often constantly. They cannot sleep, settle or sit still even for a matter of minutes. The pain and discomfort for babies is real. That I do not doubt. I have been there myself with it – twice.

I believe we should be focussing on identifying the cause of reflux and enabling you to treat that, because finding out *why* baby's tummy is doing what it's doing, and supporting their natural development feels like a better approach.

One particular statistic from the survey I carried out in 2017 tells me that medication is an international waste of money: with 60.7% of babies on medication for reflux still having symptoms, from a response population of 1,296 respondents.

This tallies with what I have observed in various online forums and with my private clients. All too often the medication does not result in a substantial improvement for baby. All too often babies are on medication – sometimes multiple – without significant results.

I asked parents of babies who were given medication to rate the positive impact that it had on their baby from 0-10, where 0 was no change

---

31 https://en.wikipedia.org/wiki/Nissen_fundoplication

in symptoms and 10 was total resolution of all symptoms. The results are astonishing.

Only 22.4% of babies experienced a dramatic improvement rated 8/10 or more. Furthermore, 21.3% of babies experience a change so small that their parents rated it 3/10 or less. These leave 56.3% of babies with some improvements, but still not complete resolution, with medications.

How Would You Rate the Impact that Medication Has Had For Your Baby?

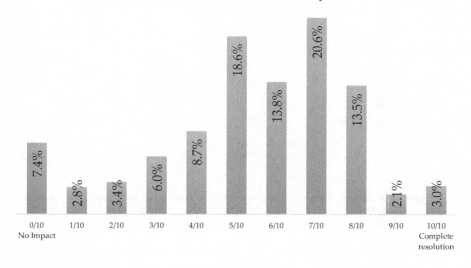

Figure 3 summaries the impact that medication has had for babies as observed by parents. Data taken from the online survey I ran between May 2017 and July 2018 with 1,499 unique responses.

On top of this, 68.2% of babies on prescription medications have tried multiple prescription medications. With so many babies on or trying multiple medications, and the medications not producing the outcomes we desire, why are we keeping our babies medicated without asking different questions?

In addition, the survey results show that 86.7% of babies diagnosed with Cow's Milk Protein Allergy (CMPA) were taking prescription medications. This is shocking because medication is not going to resolve the problem here, removing the allergen (and other potential allergens or intolerants) will have the greatest effect. The cause of the reflux is likely to be the CMPA.

If the medication isn't working so well, why are we not asking different questions? Why are parents seeking help elsewhere or changing the dose of their medications without their doctor's approval?

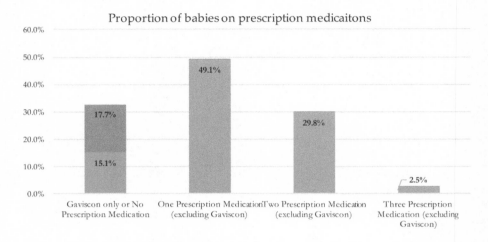

Figure 4 highlights just how frequent medication for reflux is. 81.3% of babies are on prescription medications, excluding alginates. There is a big question to ask about the frequency of medication given the effectiveness highlighted before.

Don't get me wrong. All parents are doing what they can to support their babies and stop them suffering. All parents are trying to figure it out. Most parents are getting poor support from their first port of call for help. In fact, 67.5% of parents stated they did not get adequate support when they looked for it.

I blame the culture of our healthcare providers. None, *absolutely none*, appear to be spending a little time investigating the true cause of babies' reflux. Parents are being told they are paranoid or worse. Parents are tearing their hair out because this feels awful. Parents are still not getting sleep, still having to hold down jobs, still having to bring siblings to school and function in a semi-normal way, still having to feed the family and clean the house, because all these things do not go away just because there's a reflux baby in the house.

Perhaps it's because medication is a quick answer for busy consultants. They may see high satisfaction rates because they have given parents an "answer" for what is wrong with their baby and a prescription to make everything better, which appears to be an immediate outcome. It may also be that mums are demanding medications for their babies because they are ignored so readily at first, often being told they are being paranoid and that their baby will outgrow it. Parents are not given helpful information, the next logical steps to take, or the support they need.

I know that the guidelines recommend avoiding medication in infants as much as possible.

What is missing here is the proper identification of the cause of the discomfort in the first place, and this is what I intend to change. There is no reason why babies and families should suffer for months without full and proper support. And there is no reason that babies should be left on medications, or trialling different medications to see if the next one will work.

The truth is that most parents would prefer their babies not to be on medication in the first place. But our culture is one of: something is wrong; pop a pill to fix it. I aim to change this by discovering the cause of the reflux in each case, so that we can quickly identify the best and most likely resolution for each baby.

There is absolutely a place for medications to help deal with reflux when it has been properly diagnosed, and non-medical interventions have been attempted and found to not improve or eliminate symptoms. It should be a last resort rather than the first go-to.

However, from my personal experience, I believe there is too much misdiagnosis of reflux. Daffodil was diagnosed with reflux and given prescription medication. It turned out she had a posterior tongue-tie and food allergies. Yes, she may have had reflux, but as a symptom, not the true problem. I doubt any amount of medication would have given her relief, because she would still have been drinking too much air and having allergic responses to foods unsuitable for her.

PRESCRIBING MEDICATION

When parents do get to see a consultant or GP who prescribes medication, I have found that they are typically given a prescription and dosage instructions, but little, if any, other information about the drug being prescribed. The information I believe should be given to every parent is:

- Medication name
- Active ingredient information
- How the medication works
- What impact this could have on the rest of the body
- Duration of treatment and review intervals
- Potential side effects
- Potential long-term consequences of taking the medication
- Medication weaning process.

This... as a minimum. If parents don't get this information, how can they make an informed decision? In the first instance, know that medication is not your only choice and know that there is a decision to be made. *You are the custodian of your child's health and life* until they are old enough to make their own decisions. You must be aware of any side effects and potential long-term impacts of the medications you give your child. You must weigh up the risks and benefits, and then make an informed choice about what you believe is best for your child and your family.

There are a few types of medications prescribed for reflux. These work in slightly different ways.

The reasoning behind reflux medication is that baby's stomach is "leaking" back up through the LOS into the oesophagus and causing a painful burning sensation to this sensitive tissue. In some cases of reflux, the acid can literally "burn" through the tissue causing scarring. However, this is very rare.

Medication attempts to stop or reduce the amount of acid refluxing or to neutralise the acid before it leaves the stomach to reduce potential irritation. The modalities/medications used to try to achieve these outcomes are listed below.

NOTE: Drug names are listed as the generic with the [brand] in square brackets.

Alginates (e.g. [Gaviscon]): This works by forming a gel in contact with stomach acid, with the aim of thickening the stomach contents so that they are harder to force back through the LOS. Success depends on the strength of the LOS and force of stomach "contractions". The alginate doesn't work that successfully for most babies (63.9% rating it's impact of 5/10 or less), although because it is so gentle, it is worth trying. The downside of this is that it can cause constipation. As the alginate absorbs more fluid to create the gel, there is another potential side effect: dehydration. In both cases, take great care and watch baby's fluid intake. Babies can have some water as well as milk. And if you're breastfeeding, increase your water intake too.

It can also cause hypersensitivity, gastric distension (abnormal stomach stretching and bloating, with or without pain) and bowel blockages[32]. You should not give it to your baby if they have been recommended for a low-salt diet.

Antacids (e.g. [Tums], milk of magnesia): These are an alkaline that counteracts and neutralises the stomach acid that is regurgitated, to reduce irritation to the oesophagus lining. There are relatively few prescriptions of antacids for babies so there is little information to go on regarding whether this is useful or not. However, it will not have an impact on intestinal symptoms such as wind, squirming, sleep or skin conditions. This will only address the vomiting and physical reflux symptoms.

---

32 https://www.medicines.org.uk/emc/PIL.23513.latest.pdf

Antacids can cause diarrhoea from the concentration of magnesium in them. Magnesium-containing antacids tend to be laxative, whereas aluminium-containing antacids may be constipating; antacids containing both magnesium and aluminium may reduce these colonic side effects. Aluminium accumulation can be a risk if renal function is not normal in baby.

Bismuth- and calcium-containing antacids are never recommended for infants, as the bismuth can be a neurotoxin and calcium can cause hypercalcaemia (excess calcium in the blood) and alkalosis (excessive blood alkalinity).

Histimine-2 receptor antagonists (H2RA, or H-2 blockers) (e.g. cimetidine[33] [Tagamet], ranitidine [Zantac], nizatidine [Axid], famotidine [Pepcid]): These work by stopping the histamine-2 response in the stomach and decreasing the amount of stomach acid produced. Some H-2 blockers contain other ingredients that parents should be aware may cause more discomfort to baby, such as increased wind and abdominal bloating due to the sugars not being digestible (e.g. malitol).

Proton Pump Inhibitors (PPI) (e.g. omeprazole [Prilosec, Zegerid, Omesec], lansoprazole [Prevacaid], pantoprazole [Protonix], esomeprazole [Nexium]): In brief, PPIs stop the stomach lining from producing acid by inhibiting the enzymes that trigger this mechanism.

Use of PPIs in infants increases the risk of fractures by 22%, and by 31% if they are taking an H2RA as well. The earlier the infant started on the medication, the higher their fracture risk[34].

The US Food and Drug Administration (FDA) issued various safety warnings regarding the potential effects of long-term use of PPIs including:

---

33 https://www.medicines.org.uk/emc/PIL.10429.latest.pdf
34 http://www.aappublications.org/news/2017/05/04/PASAntacids050417 Malchodi L, Apryl S, Wagner K et al. Early antacid exposure increases fracture risk in young children. Presented at the Pediatric Academic Societies Meeting; 2017 May 6-9; San Francisco, California

- Hypomagnesia (low magnesium levels in the blood)[35]
- Increased risk of fractures[36]
- Clostridium difficile – associated diarrhoea
- Vitamin B12 deficiency[37]
- Acute interstitial nephritis (AIN) (inflammation in the kidneys)
- Cutaneous and systemic lupus erythematosus events (when the immune system becomes overactive and attacks healthy tissue).

PPIs have been associated with an increased risk of vitamin and mineral deficiencies impacting vitamin B12, vitamin C, calcium, iron and magnesium metabolism[38].

Typically, these deficiencies are not addressed with any sort of supplementation in infants, because the research has not been done in the neonatal community. If these medications can affect the adult population in this manner, there is a significant likelihood that they will have similar, if not greater, effects on the immature infant.

Understanding Side Effects

"Gastric acid is an early line of defence against infection and important for the absorption of certain nutrients. Therefore, it is not surprising that adverse effects could result from suppressing acid secretion."[39]

Side effects are rated across a scale from very common to very rare. The rates for each are listed here:

Very common:	more than 1 in 10 people are affected,	more than 10%
Common:	between 1 in 10 and 1 in 100 people are affected	1% – 10%

---

35 FDA Drug Safety Communication: Low magnesium levels can be associated with long-term use of Proton Pump Inhibitor drugs (PPIs) https://www.fda.gov/drugs/drugsafety/ ucm245011.htm
36 https://www.fda.gov/drugs/drugsafety/postmarketdrugsafetyinformationforpatientsand providers/ucm213206.htm
37 https://www.fda.gov/downloads/newsevents/meetingsconferencesworkshops/ ucm495066.pdf
38 Heidelbaugh JJ. Proton pump inhibitors and risk of vitamin and mineral deficiency: evidence and clinical implications. Therapeutic Advances in Drug Safety. 2013;4(3):125-133. doi:10.1177/2042098613482484
39 http://s188618569.websitehome.co.uk/resources/PPI+use+for+reflux.pdf Journal of Paediatrics, February 2012

Uncommon:	between 1 in 100 and 1 in 1,000 people are affected	0.1% – 1%
Rare:	between 1 in 1,000 and 1 in 10,000 people are affected	0.01% – 0.1%
Very rare:	fewer than 1 in 10,000 people are affected	less than 0.01%

To be clear, when side effects are rated as "very common", they could be experienced by every person who takes that medication and still be described simply as "more than 10%" of people.

Side effects listed here are for the general medications only, which means they are applicable to all the drugs in a class.

All information about medication side effects here is taken from the UK's National Institute for Health and Care Excellence (NICE)[40] literature.

The most interesting and note-worthy part of the common or very common side effects of medications is that they are highly likely to create the exact same sorts of symptoms in the body that we are trying to relieve in our babies with reflux. Therefore, if a child is placed on medication, how could a parent be reasonably expected to tell if it is the medication causing the symptoms, ongoing reflux issues themselves or the child's normal development? In truth, you cannot tell, until you have removed the medication from the equation with sufficient time for your baby to readjust to their normal stomach acid levels.

SIDE EFFECTS FOR ALGINATES:

There are no commonly listed side effects for alginate medications, although the way in which they work would lead to a tendency for constipation. Indeed, constipation is often the reason why parents stop using alginates with their babies for reflux, as the constipation can be worse than any other previous symptoms experienced before this medication.

---

40 https://bnf.nice.org.uk

SIDE EFFECTS FOR ANTACIDS:

No side effects are available for antacids from the NICE database, although the NHS states, "Sometimes they can cause: diarrhoea or constipation; flatulence (wind); stomach cramps; feeling sick or vomiting". Unfortunately, "sometimes" is not a standard rating for drug side effects, and so we cannot tell the likely occurrence of these.

SIDE EFFECTS FOR ALL H2RA MEDICATIONS:

Common or very common: diarrhoea; dizziness; headache.

SIDE EFFECTS FOR ALL PPI MEDICATIONS:

Common or very common: abdominal pain; constipation; diarrhoea; flatulence; gastro-intestinal disturbances; headache; nausea; vomiting.

THE DANGERS OF USING MEDICATIONS

Stomach acid is natural. It is the perfect environment to support digestion, as well as acting as a first line of defence to protect our babies from bacteria or pathogens trying to enter their bodies through the digestive system. Stomach acid also contains critical digestive enzymes and is required to absorb minerals like magnesium, iron and sodium. Therefore, using medication to reduce or inhibit the production of stomach acid opens the gateway to more food and waterborne illnesses.

Research shows that the use of gastric-acid-inhibiting medications:

- Increases risk of acute gastroenteritis[42]
- Increases risk of community-acquired pneumonia[42]
- Increases incidence of intestinal and respiratory infections in otherwise healthy children, and this risk remains after the drug therapy stops[41]

---

41 Canani RB, Cirillo P, Roggero P, Romano C, Malamisura B, Terrin G, Passariello A, Manguso F, Morelli L, Guarino A; Working Group on Intestinal Infections of the Italian Society of Pediatric Gastroenterology, Hepatology and Nutrition (SIGENP).. Therapy with gastric acidity inhibitors increases the risk of acute gastroenteritis and community-acquired pneumonia in children. Pediatrics. 2006 May;117(5):e817-20. PubMed PMID: 16651285.

- Increases incidence of necrotising enterocolitis in pre-term infants[42]
- Shows higher frequency of small intestine bacteria overgrowth (SIBO) causing abdominal pain, bloating, eructation (burping), and flatulence[43]
- Increases risk of candidemia (candida fungal infection that can be fatal if not appropriately diagnosed and treated) in neonatal intensive care units[44]
- Increases occurrence of lower respiratory tract infections considered to be serious adverse events (infants, PPI)[45]
- Shows higher incidence of bone fracture in childhood after PPI use[46].

Additional consequences of using gastric-acid-inhibiting medications that have only been proven in the adult population are listed below. It may stand to reason that infants and young children exposed to these medications for prolonged periods are also likely to be at risk of:

- Bacterial overgrowth of the upper gastrointestinal tract[47]
- Increased incidence of intestinal infections[48]

---

42 Guillet R, Stoll BJ, Cotten CM, Gantz M, McDonald S, Poole WK, Phelps DL; National Institute of Child Health and Human Development Neonatal Research Network.. Association of H2-blocker therapy and higher incidence of necrotizing enterocolitis in very low birth weight infants. Pediatrics. 2006 Feb;117(2):e137-42. Epub 2006 Jan 3. PubMed PMID: 16390920

43 Sieczkowska A, Landowski P, Zagozdzon P, Kaminska B, Lifschitz C. The association of proton pump inhibitor therapy and small bowel bacterial overgrowth in children. Eur J Gastroenterol Hepatol. 2017 Oct;29(10):1190-1191. doi: 10.1097/MEG.0000000000000946. PubMed PMID: 28800034

44 Saiman L, Ludington E, Pfaller M, Rangel-Frausto S, Wiblin RT, Dawson J, Blumberg HM, Patterson JE, Rinaldi M, Edwards JE, Wenzel RP, Jarvis W. Risk factors for candidemia in Neonatal Intensive Care Unit patients. The National Epidemiology of Mycosis Survey study group. Pediatr Infect Dis J. 2000 Apr;19(4):319-24. PubMed PMID: 10783022

45 Orenstein SR, Hassall E, Furmaga-Jablonska W, Atkinson S, Raanan M. Multicenter, double-blind, randomized, placebo-controlled trial assessing the efficacy and safety of proton pump inhibitor lansoprazole in infants with symptoms of gastroesophageal reflux disease. J Pediatr. 2009 Apr;154(4):514-520.e4. doi: 10.1016/j.jpeds.2008.09.054. Epub 2008 Dec 3. PubMed PMID: 19054529

46 Yu EW, Bauer SR, Bain PA, Bauer DC. Proton pump inhibitors and risk of fractures: a meta-analysis of 11 international studies. Am J Med. 2011 Jun;124(6):519-26. doi: 10.1016/j.amjmed.2011.01.007. PubMed PMID: 21605729; PubMed Central PMCID: PMC3101476

47 Williams C, McColl KE. Review article: proton pump inhibitors and bacterial overgrowth. Aliment Pharmacol Ther. 2006 Jan 1;23(1):3-10. Review. PubMed PMID: 16393275.

48 Dial MS. Proton pump inhibitor use and enteric infections. Am J Gastroenterol. 2009 Mar;104 Suppl 2:S10-6. doi: 10.1038/ajg.2009.46. Review. PubMed PMID: 19262540.

- Nutritional deficiencies including malabsorption of vitamin B12, calcium, iron and magnesium[49] and lower serum vitamin C concentrations[50]
- Increased incidence of food allergy (animal and human data, or H2RA).

2009 clinical guidelines from both the North American Society for Pediatric Gastroenterology, Hepatology, and the Nutrition and European Society for Paediatric Gastroenterology, Hepatology, and Nutrition concluded that PPI therapy is not recommended for infants and that these drugs have little role in the management of most infants with GORD[51]. This is partly because it is difficult to tell what benefits directly come from the medication and what would happen as a normal part of ongoing development and growth.

Most proton pump inhibitor medications are ***not approved for use*** in infants under 12 months. The US FDA safety and efficacy guidelines only approve omeprazole for the treatment of GERD and not GER for up to 8 weeks in 2-16 years old only. Esomeprazole is only for ages 1 to 17 years or for the short-term use of 6 weeks for GERD only. For ranitidine (H2RA), safety and efficacy has been established for the 1-month to 16-year age group for the treatment of GERD only and should not be taken any longer than 2 weeks.

---

49 Yang YX, Metz DC. Safety of proton pump inhibitor exposure. Gastroenterology. 2010 Oct;139(4):1115-27. doi: 10.1053/j.gastro.2010.08.023. Epub 2010 Aug 19. Review. PubMed PMID: 20727892.

50 Heidelbaugh JJ. Proton pump inhibitors and risk of vitamin and mineral deficiency: evidence and clinical implications. Ther Adv Drug Saf. 2013 Jun;4(3):125-33. doi: 10.1177/2042098613482484. PubMed PMID: 25083257; PubMed Central PMCID: PMC4110863.

51 Vandenplas Y, Rudolph CD, Di Lorenzo C, Hassall E, Liptak G, Mazur L, Sondheimer J, Staiano A, Thomson M, Veereman-Wauters G, Wenzl TG, North American Society for Pediatric Gastroenterology Hepatology and Nutrition, European Society for Pediatric Gastroenterology Hepatology and Nutrition. Pediatric gastroesophageal reflux clinical practice guidelines: joint recommendations of the North American Society for Pediatric Gastroenterology, Hepatology, and Nutrition (NASPGHAN) and the European Society for Paediatric Gastroenterology, Hepatology, and Nutrition (ESPGHAN). J Pediatr Gastroenterol Nutr. 2009 Oct;49(4):498-547. doi: 10.1097/MPG.0b013e3181b7f563. PubMed PMID: 19745761

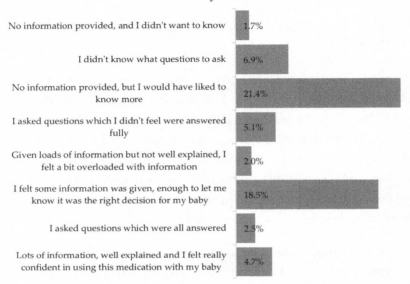

How Much Informaiton Were You Given About
Your Baby's Medication?

The information gathered in my survey indicates that about 50% of parents were inadequately prepared, or were not given as much information as they wanted or felt they needed for the medications for their baby. In addition, I observe parents frequently changing their baby's medication dose outside of the recommendations given by their GPs, without the full understanding of how these medications work or their side effects.

Could this be damaging our infant population's health for the long term? What effects will this self-medicating have on our population in 5, 10 or 30 years' time?

WEANING FROM MEDICATION

It is unfortunate that many parents are not given much information about what constitutes "long-term use", told how long to expect their child to stay on medication, or told how to wean from medication use safely and effectively.

With 77.4% of parents were give *no advice at all* about how to wean their babies from the medications and a further 16.2% of parents said it was "mentioned in passing". This is a shocking finding in that such a high proportion of prescribing doctors are not following the guidelines.

In her article for the Reflux Infants Support Association (Australia), general practitioner Dr Naomi Farragher clearly outlines how PPI medication works.

"PPIs block the acid pump which exists of the parietal cells in the lining of the stomach, stopping them from being able to pump acid from inside the cell into the stomach. The acidity of the stomach is controlled by three hormones produced by the body in response to a high (non-acidic) pH in the stomach, these hormones act on the parietal cells to make them produce more acid; however in the presence of a PPI, it cannot be moved into the stomach. It is thought that whilst on a PPI, the body produces high levels of these hormones to try and get more acid to be secreted.

When you stop using a proton pump inhibitor, at the start there will still be high levels of these hormones acting on the parietal cells getting them to make lots of acid which can now be released into the stomach. Therefore a spike in stomach acid production is inevitable."[52]

When weaning, there *will be* rebound acidosis – or a flare-up of reflux symptoms. This is unavoidable and it does not mean that your baby still has reflux. Their body needs time to readjust and regain their normal stomach acid production levels. Typically, the longer your baby has been using a gastric-acid-suppressing medication, the slower and more gradual the weaning process should be. If you currently do not have a plan for weaning from medication, it may be something you wish to speak about to your prescribing physician soon.

My clients are taught to understand how a wean can affect the foods their babies may be able to digest. The acid-suppressing medications can mask symptoms that may be present from another source, for example too

---

[52] https://www.reflux.org.au/articles/medication-tips-articles/what-every-reflux-parent-needs-to-know-about-a-medication-wean/

much air being swallowed, or incomplete breakdown and digestion of food, so take care with your baby's foods and medication wean.

Regardless of where your baby is at with food patterns, I recommend you return to a Safe Food Diet (more details in Part 3 of this book) just before the wean and maintain this diet throughout the weaning process.

THE INCREASED RISK OF DEVELOPING FOOD ALLERGIES

As we have seen, reflux medications work primarily by reducing stomach acid. This has a direct impact on baby's ability to digest food properly in the stomach, the primary organ for protein digestion. With reduced digestive ability in the stomach, partially digested proteins pass into the intestines. These partially digested proteins can trigger allergic reactions that wouldn't otherwise take place if the proteins were to be fully digested.

An allergic reaction is a reaction of the immune system. For this job, 70%[53] of the body's immune cells are in the digestive tract, where they detect and recognise potentially harmful bacteria and viruses. They do this by recognising a sequence of amino acids – or proteins. If there are amino acid combinations that look like harmful bacteria etc, immune cells launch an "attack" and this response strengthens.

By reducing stomach acid, proteins in food cannot be fully digested and the immune system in the digestive tract can mistakenly identify food substances as potentially harmful and launch the same "attack" response. When this happens, the body may associate this food stuff as a pathogen and "learn" the allergic response.

A 2013 study looking at children concluded that "treatment with GAS (gastric acid suppression) medications is associated with the occurrence of

---

53 Vighi G, Marcucci F, Sensi L, Di Cara G, Frati F. Allergy and the gastrointestinal system. Clinical and Experimental Immunology. 2008;153(Suppl 1):3-6. doi:10.1111/j.1365-2249.2008.03713.x.

food allergy."[54] In fact, there was a *367%* increase in allergies in the medicated group of children.

It is important for parents of reflux babies, especially those on medication that affect the production or constitution of stomach acid, to be more observational when introducing new foods, especially if baby has confirmed allergic responses to other food types.

4.9.3   WHEN THE DRUGS DON'T WORK

NASOGASTRIC INTUBATION FEEDING (NG TUBE)

Some babies refuse to feed due to the pain that reflux causes them. Many people believe that an infant will not starve themselves, but when instinct is faced with choices between breathing, preserving oxygen flow and avoiding pain, and feeding, the former tends to win and will take precedence over feeding.

Reflux Infants Support Association (RISA) has a good article on feed refusers[55] and strategies for managing them, Sometimes, however, a baby may need a small tube to be passed through the nose into the stomach called a nasogastric tube (NGT), or by a button through the abdominal wall directly into the stomach, to provide nutrition. RISA also has a good series of articles on tube-feeding[56].

In the case of reflux babies, the factors considered in deciding if tube-feeding is required are complex. The decision will invariably be influenced by baby's very low weight, failure to gain weight, failure to have wet nappies or bowel movements, or the appearance to be unresponsive and chronically malnourished. Another influencing factor could be if the airway is constantly being compromised by aspiration or an ineffective swallow[57].

54https://www.researchgate.net/publication/254263214_Development_of_food_allergies_in_
patients_with_Gastroesophageal_Reflux_Disease_treated_with_gastric_acid_suppressive_medications
55 http://www.reflux.org.au/articles/feeding_tips/feed-refusers-strategies-and-options/
56 http://www.reflux.org.au/articles/feeding_tips/tube-feeding-part-1/
57 http://www.reflux.org.au/articles/feeding_tips/tube-feeding-part-1/

If this is the route that your baby needs, you should have a specific individualised nutritional plan, a strategy to reduce as soon as possible and an exit plan.

Tube-feeding is often dreaded by parents, yet it can provide incredible relief to both baby and parents. Baby is no longer fighting to survive; the body can get proper nourishment and other suffering associated with reflux tends to reduce or disappear completely.

From the point of view of the parent, they no longer have the stress that baby is not getting the nourishment they need to grow and develop, and the emotional trauma of trying to convince baby to eat is taken away. It's no longer a constant battle. Parents can engage in playful activities to continue familiarising baby with food and playing with it, allowing baby to experience textures and flavours without having to swallow.

The decision to tube-feed is not one that is ever taken lightly, and is not as simple as it appears; that said, it can be life-saving and life-changing in the correct circumstances.

Many children will wean from tube-feeding successfully, learn how to eat properly and lead normal lives. There are some fabulously inspirational stories of people who have grown up and gone on to live incredibly fulfilling lives after being tube-fed.

JEJUNAL FEEDING
This is where the tube is fed directly into the small intestine and bypasses the stomach. Jejunal feeding is only considered:

- For infants who need enteral tube-feeding but who cannot tolerate intragastric feeds because of regurgitation; or
- If reflux-related pulmonary aspiration is a concern. You may observe this if your baby appears to choke a lot on regurgitated material. If you are worried about this, consult your GP immediately.

SURGERY

Nissen's fundoplication is an operation to strengthen the upper sphincter muscle of the stomach. It is done via keyhole surgery and "involves wrapping the upper part of the stomach (fundus) around the base of the oesophagus and loosely stitching it in place. This tightens the sphincter enough to reduce reflux but not so tight as to affect swallowing."[58]

It may be considered for infants and young children with severe GORD if:

- Appropriate medical treatment has been unsuccessful; or
- Feeding regimens to manage GORD prove impractical, for example, in the case of long-term, continuous, thickened enteral tube-feeding[59].

4.10   ASSOCIATED CONDITIONS & SYMPTOMS

There are several conditions that impact reflux babies that are indeed very serious. This chapter is merely to give you an awareness of what these conditions are. If you suspect your baby has any of these conditions, you **must contact your GP** straight away. If you find that you are not getting the support you want, ask for a different doctor or a referral to a specialist.

If reflux is so bad that the acid from the stomach regurgitates frequently up the back of the throat, it can irritate the structures there, causing other symptoms and problems. It is important to have an awareness of these, as treatment for symptoms alone will not resolve the reflux. Resolve the cause of the reflux and the associated symptoms should resolve also. If they are not associated with the reflux, they should be treated as separate issues and the cause of these should be identified and treated.

---

58 http://www.gosh.nhs.uk/medical-information-0/procedures-and-treatments/fundoplication
59 https://www.nice.org.uk/guidance/ng1/resources/gastrooesophageal-reflux-disease-in-children-and-young-people-diagnosis-and-management-pdf-51035086789

This section is not an exhaustive list of associated disorders, but highlights the more common effects to understand and be aware of as a parent of a reflux baby.

4.10.1   GALACTOSAEMIA

This is a very serious condition in which baby's liver cannot break down the sugar galactose properly. Lactose is a sugar molecule made from glucose and galactose. Type I galactosaemia (present from birth) can be life-threatening. Specialised feeding is required immediately. Infants present as difficult feeders, with a lack of energy, failure to gain weight, jaundice, liver damage and abnormal bleeding. It occurs in only 1 in 30,000 to 60,000 newborns[60].

4.10.2   CONGENITAL LACTASE DEFICIENCY/ALACTASIA

Lactose intolerance is not the same as an intolerance to the lactose in cow's milk. The lactose in human breastmilk is beta-lactose; that of cow's milk is alpha-lactose. Beta-lactose is broken down fully by an infant's digestive system whereas alpha-lactose is not, but rather acts as a sugar to feed the "unfriendly" bacteria in the gut. The alpha and beta refer to the types of bonds between the sugars in the milk[61].

Alactasia is when the lactase enzyme (required to break down and digest lactose sugars) is absent, leading to the small intestine not functioning as it should. It is a rare condition, and baby will have severe feeding problems, diarrhoea, vomiting and poor weight gain.

Premature infants are more prone to a deficiency of lactase: babies born at 34 weeks have only 30% lactase activity compared with full-term babies. A stool pH of 5.5 can be an indication of lactose intolerance, as there is a higher amount of lactic acid in the stool from fermented milk.

4.10.3   SECONDARY LACTOSE INTOLERANCE

Your baby may become temporarily lactose intolerant, also known as secondary lactose intolerance. This can happen when the lining of the

---

60 https://ghr.nlm.nih.gov/condition/galactosaemia
61 http://www.freedomyou.com/cows_milk_compared_to_human_milk_freedomyou.aspx

intestines has been damaged from ill-health such as a bout of diarrhoea or gastroenteritis. This will usually rectify itself within 2 to 4 weeks once your baby regains their health and the gut flora is rebuilt.

4.10.4   LARYNGOMALACIA

Literally, this means "soft larynx", and is the most common cause of stridor in infants. It is the soft and naturally immature cartilage of the upper larynx collapsing during inhalation, resulting in an airway obstruction. In rare instances, this can cause a life-threatening airway obstruction. The development of the infant means that symptoms peak at 6 months of age.

It can be recognised by sounds made during breathing:

- High-pitched sound heard on inhalation
- Coarse sounds resembling nasal congestion
- Low-pitched stertorous (laboured breathing) noises

Laryngomalacia is the most common cause of respiratory noises when infants inhale, regardless of the type of sound heard. Infants with it have a higher incidence of reflux. In reflux babies, laryngomalacia is sometimes associated with symptoms including choking and gagging. Sounds begin around 4 to 6 weeks of age, peak by about 6 to 8 months and resolve by 2 years[62].

Most cases are mild and should be reviewed and monitored regularly. In some instances, surgery may be appropriate depending on the severity of the stridor. Appropriateness of surgery is assessed if the baby's airway becomes too obstructed and/or if feeding difficulties present such that normal growth is prevented. In some cases, where the laryngomalacia is causing obstructive sleep apnoea, pressure-assisted ventilation may be used.

---

62 https://emedicine.medscape.com/article/1002527-overview

Further information on how to differentiate between mild, moderate and severe laryngomalacia can be found on the British Medical Journal Best Practice website[63].

4.10.5   STRIDOR

Stridor is a high-pitched wheezing sound caused by disrupted airflow. Airflow is usually disrupted by a blockage in the larynx (voice box) or trachea (windpipe). Stridor is an observable symptom rather than a disease or illness itself. As a symptom, it is important to be able to identify if your baby has this.

Your baby may exhibit stridor breathing continuously or not. You may observe that lying in certain positions aggravate or alleviate it. Its presence on more than one occasion is important to report to your baby's GP. There may be something underlying the stridor that requires investigation, monitoring and/or treatment. Stridor is a red flag symptom that indicates difficulty breathing.

4.10.6   SANDIFER'S SYNDROME

Sandifer's Syndrome is often observed and described as "bizarre head and neck movements" of an infant. These movements are abnormal and dystonic. A dystonic movement is one caused by muscle spasms and contractions. They are often repetitive and cause unusual, awkward postures. They are sometimes accompanied by sudden or jerky eye movements. Sandifer's Syndrome is not dystonia, in which these movements have a neurological pathology.

A critical point for diagnosing Sandifer's rather than a neurological issue is that brain electrical activity monitoring during an episode returns normal results. Patients with Sandifer's Syndrome are "often misdiagnosed due to their paroxysmal neurobehaviours, and they receive unnecessary medication". The abnormal posturing associated with this syndrome may

---

63 http://bestpractice.bmj.com/best-practice/monograph/754/treatment/step-by-step.html

be the result of extreme sensitivity of the oesophagus to refluxed gastric acid[64] regardless of its cause (for example, too much air or an allergy).

If the infant has been accurately diagnosed as having reflux or an allergy that results in Sandifer's, then properly treating the *cause* of the reflux will resolve the condition.

There is a danger that infants presenting with the dystonic movements may be misdiagnosed and receive unnecessary medication. Medication that will not help their situation; it does not treat for the cause of the Sandifer's. There are subsequent knock-on effects of the long-term use of medications that are not needed, along with all the possible side effects they may bring with them.

While Sandifer's is relatively benign, it is a symptom of something else. If the cause is not properly treated, then it could result in torticollis and or hiatus hernia.

4.10.7   HOARSE VOICE & REFLUX LARYNGITIS
A hoarse voice is caused by swelling and mucus in the back of the voice box. In a study from 2000, 70% of children with hoarse voice aged 2-12 were identified as having a pathological GOR[65]. A hoarse voice is symptomatic of reflux laryngitis where the voice box has become inflamed due to the presence of regurgitated acid from the stomach.

4.10.8   COUGH
Cough from chronic irritation of the larynx and bronchus can occur when stomach acid reaches this point and irritates the nerve endings. This is often a dry or itchy cough.

The epithelial cells (lining of the tubes) of the respiratory system act like guards to a castle, and secrete mucus to protect the respiratory system.

---

64 http://onlinelibrary.wiley.com/resolve/openurl?genre=article&sid=nlm:pubmed&issn=0012-1622&date=1980&volume=22&issue=3&spage=374

65 https://www.ncbi.nlm.nih.gov/pubmed/?term=ssessment+of+gastroesophageal+reflux+in+the+course+of+chronic+hoarseness+in+children

When acid reaches the back of the throat, these cells produce mucus to protect the respiratory system from stomach acid. The result is a productive cough.

The epithelial cells of the digestive system produce mucus to lubricate for the movement of food, protect the stomach walls from stomach acid and filter out dirt, pollen and other microscopic particles to protect the body.

4.10.9   SUBGLOTTIC STENOSIS

This is an abnormal narrowing of the subglottis, an area of the windpipe just below the vocal cords. It can be present at birth (congenital subglottic stenosis) or develop later, typically after damage or injury; this can be because of an infection or reflux. It has the potential to happen quickly causing a life-threatening airway blockage and so is important to recognise. A key and common symptom is stridor. Others include shortness of breath, failure to thrive and recurrent episodes of croup.

4.10.10   ENLARGED ADENOIDS

Children with reflux can also have enlarged tonsils and/or adenoids. The lymphatic system is a major part of the body's immune system. It helps the body get rid of anything it identifies as a toxin, waste or otherwise unwanted material. Lymph nodes can become swollen and irritated by acid regurgitation in response to a food that the body sees as an irritant.

A study was conducted in 2001 that compared children under 2 who had enlarged adenoids (symptomatic adenoid hypertrophy) that required surgical removal (AD group) with a group who had glue ear (otitis media with effusion) needing a ventilation tube inserted without removing the adenoids (VT group).

It was seen that 42% of children under 2 having their adenoids removed had reflux disease compared with only 7% in the VT group; where the children were under 12 months of age, the incidence of reflux disease was

88%[66]. This indicates a strong link between reflux (or silent reflux) and enlarged adenoids. In addition, there is recent research linking adenoid inflammation with local allergies[67]. Could the adenoids be an indicator of allergy or intolerance which is causing the reflux?

The knock-on impact of this is that children are often identified as requiring a removal of adenoids and tonsils, which will not address the problem. It does not address the reflux or resolve that at root cause.

Additionally, it removes the body's primary signalling system that something is not as it should be. The adenoids are especially important for young children as their lymphatic system is underdeveloped at birth. They represent the first line of defence to viruses, bacteria and other pathogens ingested by breathing or eating.

4.10.11   RHINOSINUSITIS (NOSE & SINUS INFECTIONS)

In truth, rhinosinusitis is not an infection, but presents just like nose and sinus infections do. It is an inflammation of nasal passages and sinus cavities. The inflammation can be simply because of regurgitated acid at the back of the throat. Often mistaken as a cold or illness, this will not respond to any drugs because the cause is not bacterial (or viral). It will present as an ongoing and chronic condition and may change in severity due to diet.

I have found in my practice that this symptom is more frequently indicative of an allergy or food intolerance rather than being the result of acid irritation, although both can occur.

---

66 Carr, M. M., Poje, C. P., Ehrig, D. and Brodsky, L. S. (2001), Incidence of Reflux in Young Children Undergoing Adenoidectomy. The Laryngoscope, 111: 2170–2172. doi:10.1097/00005537-200112000-00018 https://www.ncbi.nlm.nih.gov/pubmed/11802019

67 Zhang X, Sun B, Li S, Jin H, Zhong N, Zeng G. Local atopy is more relevant than serum sIgE in reflecting allergy in childhood adenotonsillar hypertrophy. Pediatr Allergy Immunol 2013: 24: 422–426. https://www.ncbi.nlm.nih.gov/pubmed/23724785

4.10.12　NECROTISING ENTEROCOLITIS

This is a serious condition in which the tissues in the gut become inflamed and start to die. It can be life-threatening if not treated and occurs most commonly in pre-term infants. Common symptoms include bloating, abdominal swelling, bloody stools and diarrhoea.

NEC is a risk factor due to the use of strong acid-blocking medications such as H2 blockers and PPI[68]. It is also associated with formula-fed pre-term infants[69].

4.10.13　PYLORIC STENOSIS

This is a condition that blocks the stomach contents from moving into the small intestine. It affects the pylorus muscle at the bottom of the stomach rather than the top (as in the majority of reflux cases). It occurs in about 3 in every 1,000 live births (0.3% of babies).

Babies often present as reflux disease cases, with projectile vomiting and other reflux symptoms. Unusual symptoms that you do not see in reflux are stomach contractions before vomiting that can be observed externally as a rippling across the abdomen. Babies will not gain weight and may lose weight. The milk they vomit will be curdled as it stays in the stomach for a long time. These babies will pass very little stool, since little or no food reaches the bowel.

It tends to present by 6 weeks of age and affects boys more than girls. An operation is required to rectify and is very successful, almost

---

Zhang X, Sun B, Li S, Jin H, Zhong N, Zeng G. Local atopy is more relevant than serum sIgE in reflecting allergy in childhood adenotonsillar hypertrophy. Pediatr Allergy Immunol 2013: 24: 422–426.

https://www.ncbi.nlm.nih.gov/pubmed/23724785" https://www.ncbi.nlm.nih.gov/pubmed/23724785

Science. Advances in Neonatal Care. 2012;12(2):77-89. doi:10.1097/ANC.0b013e31824cee94.

immediately stopping vomiting after feeds[70]. It is important to diagnose this as babies can become quickly dehydrated with recurrent vomiting.

4.11   SUMMARY

So far, we've seen the well-known path of reflux and the sorts of options you might expect to hear about if you have a reflux baby, right through to some of the most serious options for severe cases.

As you know by now, my own approach focuses on food and diet individualised to you and your baby, whose immature digestive system is not coping.

The rest of this book is dedicated to explaining more about babies' digestion and what you can try to support baby's digestive health, tackling reflux at the root cause, with the aim of seeing a turnaround in your child's unsettledness and pain.

---

70 http://www.gosh.nhs.uk/medical-information/pyloric-stenosis

PART 2

UNDERSTANDING
REFLUX BABIES

5   Anatomy That Impacts Life

5.1   Give Baby a Chance

In today's world, we seem obsessed with babies' development. What they should be doing by when and how. We tend to forget about the journey their bodies need to go on.

We all know that infancy is the fastest rate of growth and change in a person's entire life. We have the books, the videos, the apps for seeing what cognitive development is going on, what physical development is happening. We get worried if our friend's baby can roll over before ours can walk. We compare our children to one other. We question what our child is and is not doing. And while all this has a place because it is helpful to understand development, we completely miss the internal physiological development and growth that our children must go through.

We rush them. We ignore the *immense* changes their bodies are going through and what needs to happen for such changes to occur. Judging from the way we feed our children by the time they are just 6 months old, it appears we are expecting their bodies to be up to speed and ready to feed naturally.

Stop and think for a moment. By the time any baby is born, they have spent 9 months growing from a single cell. For the entire time in-utero, baby has been fed by the placenta, 100% passively on their part. When baby is born, they go through what is probably the biggest shock of their lives...

When all they've ever known was ripped from them in a surge of pressure and force, baby was unprepared for it; ready for it, of course, because the accommodation was getting a bit cramped in there, but baby was still warm, cosy and not hungry.

Suddenly... Bright lights! Clear sounds much louder than before! A prickly feeling on the skin! I can feel my skin. What is this stuff? It's all over me. I'm cold. Now I'm being wrapped up in something. Oh that's good... I can smell her, my mother. There she is. Whatever else is happening, mummy is here. I will be okay. But there's a strange feeling somewhere in my body, between my head and my toes, it's empty. I'm empty. I need something. There's mummy again. And what's this beside my mouth? I think I need to do something with this. I'm not sure what, but this feels good, this feels yummy...

Think about all the processes that baby must go through, everything baby must figure out in the first few minutes of life.

As a culture, we neglect to consider what baby experiences. But there's an alternative. We can remember. I fell into **gentle parenting** and **attached parenting** because I trusted myself. And I started to understand and take stock of the scale of development that was needed for my baby.

When born, babies have a suck-swallow reflex that supports nutrition. The stomach serves mostly as a place to activate gastric-lipase and start fat digestion. Their digestive process is supported by the mother's breastmilk, so if bottle-fed, baby is reliant on his small intestine to complete the digestion of milk. This can result in incomplete digestion as formula milks do not have digestive enzymes in them to complement and support the developing digestive system.

With growth, development and time, your baby's body develops the ability to produce different enzymes in response to different food stimuli. This response process grows and develops *gradually* and is unique to every child.

5.2   BABY'S DIGESTIVE SYSTEM

The digestive system starts at the mouth, includes the oesophagus, stomach, pancreas, small intestine and large intestine. Not until all the elements of this system are mature can children be considered to have a digestive system comparable to adults. We have overlooked this important part of development, and this may be impacting the cognitive development of our children and indeed their lifelong health. It also plays a role in allergic reactions, childhood obesity and illnesses.

Most of the literature available about childhood development focuses on studies of brain and cognitive development at infancy. There is a massive piece missing in the research... the *entire body* is underdeveloped at birth in a newborn compared to most other species. We can see this clearly on the physical side: baby animals walk within minutes of being born. We know that human babies are born underdeveloped, underdeveloped by at least half the development stage of a newborn chimpanzee.

"Indeed, by one estimation a human foetus would have to undergo a gestation period of 18 to 21 months instead of the usual 9 to be born at a neurological and cognitive development stage comparable to that of a chimpanzee newborn."[71]

However, what about internal development, not just cognitive, which vitally includes the digestive system? We know that the infant digestive system "is significantly different from a miniature version of the adult digestive system"[72] in terms of its functionality and maturity.

Infants are born with a gut permeability greater than that of a healthy adult. This means that larger nutritional molecules can be absorbed more effectively by a newborn[73]. The reason for this is to increase the absorption of nutrients from milk. This is *normal stage* of development for an infant, because their gut needs to be able to absorb nutrients from mother's milk as fast as possible. However, it can cause problems if the gut absorbs undigested proteins that are then recognised by the body as a pathogen, as

71 https://blogs.scientificamerican.com/observations/why-humans-give-birth-to-helpless- babies/
72 Abrahamse E, Minekus M, van Aken GA, et al. Development of the Digestive System—Experimental Challenges and Approaches of Infant Lipid Digestion. Food Digestion. 2012;3(1-3):63-77. doi:10.1007/s13228-012-0025-x.
73 van Elburg RM, Fetter WPF, Bunkers CM, et al Intestinal permeability in relation to birth weight and gestational and postnatal age Archives of Disease in Childhood – Fetal and Neonatal Edition 2003;88:F52-F55.

this can stimulate an allergic response by the immune system, as explained in Part 1.

This image summarises (the detail of which follows in a table) how immature your baby's digestive system is in the early months of life, and why I believe that a more gentle approach to introducing foods is required.

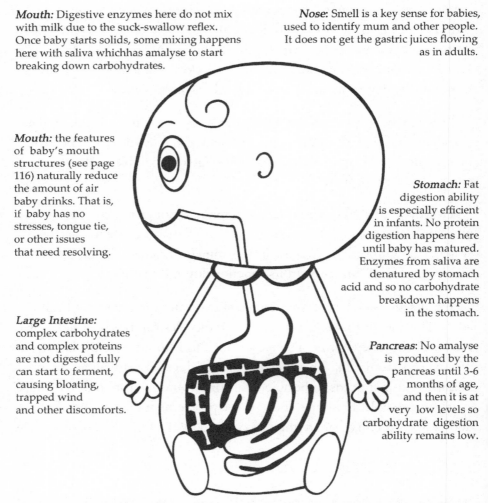

Mouth: Digestive enzymes here do not mix with milk due to the suck-swallow reflex. Once baby starts solids, some mixing happens here with saliva whichhas amalyse to start breaking down carbohydrates.

Nose: Smell is a key sense for babies, used to identify mum and other people. It does not get the gastric juices flowing as in adults.

Mouth: the features of baby's mouth structures (see page 116) naturally reduce the amount of air baby drinks. That is, if baby has no stresses, tongue tie, or other issues that need resolving.

Stomach: Fat digestion ability is especially efficient in infants. No protein digestion happens here until baby has matured. Enzymes from saliva are denatured by stomach acid and so no carbohydrate breakdown happens in the stomach.

Large Intestine: complex carbohydrates and complex proteins are not digested fully can start to ferment, causing bloating, trapped wind and other discomforts.

Pancreas: No amalyse is produced by the pancreas until 3-6 months of age, and then it is at very low levels so carbohydrate digestion ability remains low.

Small Intestine: infants have about 10% their adult level of carbohydrate digetive enzyme and about 90% of their protein digestive enzyme levels. Complex proteins that are not partially digested by stomach acid before reacting the small intestine can be mis-interpreted by the body as pathogens / allergens

Part of Digestive System	Infant Characteristics or Response
Sensory – thought, sight and smell of food	No responses measured in infants. Likely that the overall sensory system is too immature to stimulate a response from sight.
	Infants are known to understand smell of breastmilk and smell of mother, so this may well play an important role in preparing the digestive system for food on the way.
Mouth – tongue	Your baby's mouth structures are significantly different from yours – try sucking on a bottle and see how difficult it is! This is because the shape of your mouth is so different.
	Sucking and swallowing are reflexes at birth. Tongue thrust reflex is present to prevent the infant swallowing anything not associated with the suck-swallow reflex. This is to support the sucking action needed to get milk.
	See Figure 5 for more details on infant oral structures.
	Produces salivary amylase, but "no digestion of starches occurs in the mouth or oesophagus during the first months of life"[74] unlike an adult.
	Lingual lipase is secreted at the back of the tongue and starts to break down milk fats in the stomach.
Stomach	At birth, your baby's stomach is tiny, about 5-7ml or 1.5 teaspoons. Importantly, at this stage, it does not stretch. This grows rapidly to about 150ml by the age of 1 month. At 6 months, it is about 250ml and your baby's tummy size at rest is about that of their clenched fist.
	It then follows the growth trajectory of the body, like an adult's. It now stretches with food, but don't over-stretch; watch out for signs from baby to indicate fullness.
	Detailed quantitative information about the infant digestive process in the stomach is limited, but it is understood to be as follows:
	Protein digestion in the stomach is "extremely limited", but is supported by intestinal protein digestion. The stomach can secrete hydrochloric acid, and concentrations of pepsin (the enzyme for protein digestion) are low and increase over the first few months of life. Little, if any, breakdown of proteins is done by the stomach in infants. Complex proteins like casein need stomach pepsin to start the digestive process that can then be completed in the small intestine. This does not happen in infants and can lead baby's body to see casein

---

74 Akre, James, ed. "Physiological Development of the Infant and Its Implications for Complementary Feeding." *Bulletin of the World Health Organization* 67. Suppl (1989): 55–67.

Part of Digestive System	Infant Characteristics or Response
	as an allergen, leading to CMPA that baby may later grow out of with normal development.
	Fat is "quantitatively much more significant than in adults" because of an increased amount of gastric lipase[75]. Fat digestion is considerably aided by the presence of lipase contained within human breastmilk, which also supports the absorption of vitamin A.
	Starch is not digested in the stomach. The stomach acid pH level stops the amylase from saliva working. Starch is better digested by breastfed infants because of additional amylase they receive from breastmilk.
Gastrointestinal tract	Originally thought to be sterile at birth, our little babies are teeming with bacteria at birth from the placenta. The microbiome of the placenta is closest to the human oral microbiome in make-up.
	However, more significant gut microbiome development is induced by birth, with a massive colonisation of bacteria from mum. Vaginal birth, in particular, provides specific bacterium that promote ongoing positive gut microbiome development[76].
	Breastmilk continues to promote the colonisation and maturing of the infant's gut bacteria.
Small intestine	Term infants have about 10% of adult levels of amylase activity in the small intestine. Pancreatic amylase is not produced until at least 3 months of age. "It has been found to be present only at very low levels, or absent altogether, up to 6 months of age…Undigested starches may interfere with the absorption of other nutrients and result in failure to thrive in infants, and can also cause gastrointestinal problems and diarrhoea. These compensatory, or complementary mechanisms for fat utilization are less efficient when cow's-milk fat or other fats are introduced into the young infant's diet."[77]

---

75 Digestion in the newborn. Hamosh M1. Department of Pediatrics, Georgetown University Medical Center, Washington, DC, USA. Clin Perinatol. 1996 Jun;23(2):191-209.

76 https://www.ncbi.nlm.nih.gov/pmc/articles/PMC4464665/ Mueller NT, Bakacs E, Combellick J, Grigoryan Z, Dominguez-Bello MG. The infant microbiome development: mom matters. Trends in molecular medicine. 2015;21(2):109-117. doi:10.1016/j.molmed.2014.12.002.

77 Akre, James, ed. Infant Feeding: The Physiological Basis. Bulletin of the World Health Organisation, Supplement to Vol.67, 1989, P. 56-67

http://apps.who.int/iris/bitstream/10665/39084/1/bulletin_1989_67%28supp%29.pdf?ua=1

Part of Digestive System	**Infant Characteristics or Response**
	Pancreatic lipase and bile salts are very low in the newborn. Fat digestion is supported by breastmilk, comparable with the adult concentration, and thus the infant can digest most proteins.
	The lining of the small intestine has a greater permeability and can allow large molecules to pass into circulation. Undigested protein molecules can be absorbed and this can trigger an antibody response, e.g. an allergic reaction to the proteins. For this reason, careful selection of proteins in the first months of feeding is important, as is the make-up of a breastfeeding mother's diet and gut health.

Your baby's naturally immature digestive system needs to be treated with gentle care and respect in the first 2 years of life until it has naturally developed into a more mature stage. This is outwardly recognisable by observing the most obvious demonstration of the digestive system from baby – their teeth!

When we examine the structure of the mouth and throat of infants compared to that of adults, there are some distinctive differences that impact infants' needs.

This illustration overleaf of a section through an infant's head shows a number of important physiological structures that I think it is important for us, as parents, to understand a little more.

- Your baby's tongue is relatively larger in respect to the overall mouth cavity when compared with an adults' tongue and mouth; and the "free space" in the mouth is small. This supports breastfeeding and the removal of air from the mouth when drinking milk.
- The roof of baby's mouth is different: the upper palate is flat; the soft palate is large. This is the opposite to those of an adult. The soft palate is primarily muscle which supports breastfeeding.

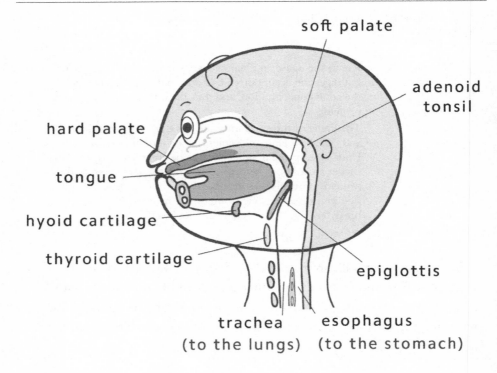

soft palate

adenoid
tonsil

hard palate

tongue

hyoid cartilage

thyroid cartilage

epiglottis

trachea   esophagus
(to the lungs) (to the stomach)

Figure 5 shows a cross section of an infants head detailing the mouth structures important for feeding, breathing and understanding reflux. An infant's tongue in relation to their mouth is much larger relative to an adult's tongue in an adult mouth, and the free space in the mouth is small. The upper palate is flat. The soft palate is large. The hyoid cartilage is close to the middle of the underside of the tongue. The epiglottis and thyroid cartilage are close together. The oesophagus is narrow

- The position of the epiglottis (the "flap" that shuts off the windpipe when swallowing to ensure food goes down the oesophagus) is significantly different, with it virtually touching the soft palate in the infant. Again, this supports the liquid-only diet of the infant and reduces the risk of drowning. With the suck-swallow reflex, the epiglottis appears to close and protect the airway in an infant when swallowing. There is no opening to allow milk held in the mouth to "leak" into the airway.

- Worthy of note is that the adenoids are significantly larger in the infant than the adult. This is because as the beginning of the development of the lymphatic system, they have an important role in trapping pathogens to protect the infant's body. As part of the lymphatic system, adenoids can also become inflamed in response to a food substance that the body does not tolerate well[78].

All these differences between the baby and human mouth structures are significant from a feeding point of view – baby has a much greater risk of choking on foods when introduced due to the narrower airway.

Moving down the digestive system, the oesophagus is the tube that connects the mouth to the stomach. In infants with problematic reflux, the length of the abdominal oesophagus is significantly shorter than infants without. The shorter the oesophagus, the more severe the reflux experienced[79]. The oesophagus elongates as part of normal development, yet every child is different, and so is their growth trajectory. What this tells us is that, as we know, children *will* grow out of reflux, but you cannot put a time on it.

Oesophagus length may also indicate when a baby will be ready to wean from medication. Of course, these questions need much greater scientific study, but we can keep this information in the back of our minds when considering baby's readiness for weaning from medication.

The stomach, the organ thought of as the powerhouse of the digestive system, is next in line. The food mixed with saliva in the mouth continues to have its sugars broken down by salivary amylase. The greater the mixing of food and saliva in the mouth, the greater the breakdown of carbohydrates in this part of the digestive system. This is important, because once food enters the stomach, stomach acid stops the action of amylase, by between 50% and 100% depending on what else is in the food.

---

78 Zhang X, Sun B, Li S, Jin H, Zhong N, Zeng G. Local atopy is more relevant than serum sIgE in reflecting allergy in childhood adenotonsillar hypertrophy. Pediatr Allergy Immunol. 2013 Aug;24(5):422-6. doi: 10.1111/pai.12089. Epub 2013 Jun 3. PubMed PMID: 23724785.

79 Sonographic measurement of the abdominal esophagus length in infancy: a diagnostic tool for gastroesophageal reflux. Koumanidou C1, Vakaki M, Pitsoulakis G, Anagnostara A, Mirilas P. AJR Am J Roentgenol. 2004 Sep;183(3):801-7

For parents, it is vital to understand what the digestive system can and cannot break down so that we can take it into consideration when feeding our child.

5.2.1   GAS/WIND

Gas, or wind, is completely normal. It happens to us all. What is important is the smell, as this is a giveaway of what is going on inside.

There are typically two types of gas: the smelly stuff and the not-so-smelly stuff. Both occur naturally but for different reasons. Smelly gas can be the result of fermentation in the gut and can indicate improper digestion, irritation of the gut itself by specific foods, or a microbial imbalance. Non-smelly gas is typically air that is swallowed. This can be swallowed when babies feed or cry, or when older babies and children talk or laugh. As you can see, many of these sources of air are also completely normal.

Internal air becomes a problem when it is present in excess and causes pain or discomfort of some kind, or when the body is constipated, which causes air to build up and not pass easily.

If baby has excessive wind, trapped or painful wind, or smelly wind, it could be an indication of any of the following[80]:

- Improper digestion (due to totally natural immaturity of baby's gut)
- Food sensitivities
- Fermentation of food in the gut
- Constipation
- Excessive bacteria in the small intestine
- Too much air being consumed for a variety of reasons.

---

80 https://draxe.com/flatulence/

5.3   Breastfeeding

Breastmilk is magical. And I don't say that lightly. I understand that some women cannot breastfeed for various reasons, and to these ladies, my heart goes out. I know several incredible women who have moved hell and high water to provide breastmilk for their newborns. For those who wish to breastfeed and cannot, I respect you and your strength.

Breastfeed if you can. If you really want to do what's best for your baby, get over your faux-phobia and do what baby needs! No more: "Ugh! That grosses me out!" This was me! For those of you who choose not to, I respect your right to choose and encourage you to make sure you make an informed choice.

A study in *The Lancet* in 2016 stated, "The decision not to breastfeed has major long-term negative effects on the health, nutrition and development of children and on women's health."[81] There is no doubt that breastfeeding is the best option for mum and baby. I believe in choice, yet part of the choice to have a baby is the acceptance of the responsibility for that child, including provision of the best nutritional start possible.

5.3.1   Breastfeeding: My Story

During my pregnancy, I didn't think much about what I would do when baby actually arrived. I was a fly-by-the-seat-of-my-pants sort and felt everything would just be okay. I had great plans about how my baby would be in a great routine, how she'd be sleeping through by 12 weeks, and how wonderful life would be. The truth was far from this.

When it came to breastfeeding, I hadn't given it much thought either, except that I would try and see how far I got. I believed in the benefits that breastfeeding would give my baby. I wanted her to have the best start in life. I didn't attend any breastfeeding courses when pregnant. I sort of assumed it would come naturally.

81http://www.thelancet.com/series/maternal-and-child-nutrition

When my little girl was born, she latched beautifully. I was lucky. And yes, it felt a little weird, but to be honest, being pregnant had freaked me out too! Once I decided I would feed her, I was determined to put up with the pain and sleepless nights, and do my best. With a reflux baby, it meant many feeds, many times a night, every night.

With my first baby, we both had severe pain at the start, which I was told was normal. She was 6 weeks old before I asked for help. I knew Sunflower was gaining weight nicely, and breastfeeding had become more comfortable. Nonetheless, I went along to a breastfeeding clinic with a friend. Mainly as support for her, but the truth was I needed it too. Within 10 minutes, the lactation consultant tweaked my baby's position and the change was drastic in terms of comfort. But it didn't change our nights.

A baby's body absorbs every ounce of goodness possible. My second baby Daffodil had a bowel movement only every 10 days! I am serious! I took her to the doctor several times, worried she wasn't having regular bowel movements. After much reassurance from my GP, midwives, health visitors, all of whom did exclaim it was a long time to go between, she was fine. As long as Daffodil was having plenty of wet nappies and drinking enough milk, she'd be okay. After a few months of this, I realised that my daughter was, in fact, having a regular bowel movement, regular being every 10 days! And I didn't complain any longer. I could go for 10 days safe in the knowledge that there wouldn't be an explosion to cope with!

I started to reframe "normal" for myself. I realised that my diet was so clean and nutritionally dense that baby's body was absorbing virtually everything she drank. I used hindsight to reinforce this; once Daffodil started eating real food, it was virtually like a switch was turned on and she started having daily bowel movements.

5.3.2   SO HOW DOES BREASTFEEDING WORK?

A mother's diet directly influences breastmilk, and therefore, the nutrition baby gets and needs. There is a responsive mechanism at work between mother and baby. Mother's body can detect, through a feedback loop, what baby needs at any given time, and alter the composition of the milk to support her baby.

According to La Leche League's description of diffusion, anything that a mum consumes, breathes or applies to her skin has the potential to get into her breastmilk via her bloodstream.

Every lactating woman, therefore, ought to have an awareness of her environment, diet and skincare. Why is this important for breastfeeding mums? Because if you have a truly unsettled baby, you need to look at the combination of environmental, dietary, medical and skincare information with that of the maturity of your baby's digestive system and what it can handle. You must have this awareness of when feeding baby, especially an unsettled baby.

This transfer of substances from the breastfeeding mother's environment and diet to the infant is more pronounced in mums who have a syndrome called "leaky gut", which is common and worth covering briefly here.

5.3.3   WHAT IS LEAKY GUT?

Leaky gut syndrome, or increased intestinal permeability, is when the lining of the large intestine is inflamed and the 'holes' that allow nutritional elements to pass the intestinal barrier are essentially enlarged. This allows nutrients to pass into the blood, but also lets bigger-than-usual particles "leak" into the bloodstream. These particles that ordinarily wouldn't be in the bloodstream can cause various imbalances in how your body operates. As we know, anything that gets into your blood can get into your breastmilk. Equally, the particles have the potential to cause various imbalances in how baby's body operates too.

With complex sugars, molecules can cross your gut barrier and get into your milk. That means there is a high likelihood that these sugars will be causing your baby a problem, because they are simply not mature enough to be equipped to break them down. As a result, they ferment in your baby's system causing abdominal discomfort.

With proteins, intact protein molecules can pass into your circulatory system and then your milk. As baby has limited protein digestion, these whole protein molecules pass into baby's circulation and can result in an allergic reaction.

5.3.4   LEAKY GUT: HOW TO TELL

So how do you know if you have a leaky gut? According to Mind Body Green[82], the following are leaky gut symptoms. You may only have one symptom or you may have many:

1. Food allergies, intolerances or sensitivities, or nutritional deficiencies
2. Digestive issues such as gas, bloating, diarrhoea, constipation, IBS or Crohn's disease
3. Headaches, brain fog, poor concentration, memory loss
4. Sinusitis or rhinitis
5. Seasonal allergies or asthma
6. Hormonal imbalances like PMS or PCOS
7. Autoimmune diseases such as rheumatoid arthritis, Hashimoto's thyroiditis, lupus, or coeliac disease
8. Excessive fatigue, chronic fatigue or fibromyalgia
9. Mood and mind issues like depression, anxiety, ADD or ADHD
10. Skin conditions like acne, rosacea, psoriasis or eczema
11. Weakened immune system
12. Thyroid conditions
13. Sugar or carb cravings.

If mum has a leaky gut, increased gut permeability or a localised inflammation in her gut, partially digested food particles (proteins and or sugars) can reach her blood stream. If the particles are small enough to cross the intestine-blood barrier, they are probably small enough to cross the barrier from blood to breastmilk. Baby doesn't have the digestive maturity, the correct enzymes to break down these food particles. The food therefore irritates the gut when it gets there.

---

82 https://www.mindbodygreen.com/0-10908/9-signs-you-have-a-leaky-gut.html

- So often, this irritation is the pain baby is feeling when we speak of "reflux".
- Sugars ferment in baby's gut causing excess gas that their system is not yet mature enough to pass.
- This causes discomfort and further pain.
- Proteins that require high levels of stomach pH are not digested enough in baby's stomach and move into the gut, also causing irritation and pain.

If you are a breastfeeding mum and think you might have a leaky gut, your food could be having a great impact on your baby, resulting in a reflux diagnosis, but there is more to the story... It may be fully resolved by modifying what and how you eat. From personal experience of having this, I could see the impact of my food on my baby. I witnessed a direct correlation between food and symptoms with both my children.

5.3.5   DEALING WITH AN UNSETTLED BREASTFED BABY

If your baby is generally unsettled, know that you don't have to stop breastfeeding. I suggest you **keep breastfeeding**, because so often I hear mothers have been advised that their milk is causing the reflux and to quit. Remember, your baby *cannot* be allergic to your breastmilk.

First and foremost, if you are struggling, please, please, please, find an IBCLC and get support. While breastfeeding is natural, it does not come naturally – it is a skill to be learned and there are lots of really good teachers out there. You do not have to do it alone, the support could make a world of difference.

As a breastfeeding mum, do as much as possible to rebuild your own gut health, identify and avoid irritants for you, and continue to look after your baby.

You can ensure you have good bacteria by eating prebiotic foods, such as broccoli and cauliflower. You can reduce the stimulation of bad bacteria by reducing your sugar intake, which is also a good idea to support your baby's digestive system because they cannot digest sugar until about 2 years of age.

You can rebuild your gut health by taking a suitable probiotic supplement. Select a probiotic carefully, in case your baby has CMPA, as many probiotics are derived from cow's milk and are not suitable for babies with CMPA. You can also eat fermented foods (dairy-free, if necessary), such as kimchi and homemade sauerkraut, to restore your gut to full health.

Changing your diet can have a marked impact on your baby's unsettled behaviour. To find out what impacts baby most, I suggest my elimination diet, and a strict food and symptom diary for a few weeks to see what makes a difference. The details are in Section 10 The Breastfeeding Protocol (page 199).

6   WHAT'S IN BABY'S MILK?

Let's go on and look at formula milks for babies. Whether baby is on formula by mum's choice, medical issues or reflux, the fact is bottle-feeding may be where you're at right now. I want to do everything I can to support you and provide you with as much information about the milks out there, so you can understand potential issues. The bottom line is some milks might work better for some babies and other milks might be favourable for other babies.

Although I can't cover every formula milk on the market within the scope of this book, this chapter teaches you how to read the labels and ingredients to have a greater understanding of what is in the milk. This will give you a better chance of identifying what might be working or not for your child. The most important point to remember is that every child and every digestive system is *different*; what works for one may not work for the next.

6.1   FORMULA MILKS

Not all formula milks are created equal. There are significant differences, but by combining your current knowledge of baby's symptoms and what those symptoms may indicate, pick a milk you think is best to try, and have an awareness of what to watch.

6.1.1   COW'S MILK FORMULA (STANDARD FORMULA)

Most infant formula milks are based on cow's milk, which is meant for baby cows. Cows have a completely different digestive process to humans. Simple physiology tells us this: cow stomachs have four chambers, meaning extensive stomach digestion. Humans have a single stomach chamber. Therefore, the balance of proteins, fats and carbohydrates in cow's milk needs to be manually (artificially) adjusted to make it suitable for human babies.

Common additives to cow's-milk-based formulas include iron and vitamins to meet nutritional needs.

6.1.2   ANTI-REGURGITATION/THICKENED FORMULA

Anti-regurgitation (AR) formulas are often referred to as anti-reflux milks. You might think to try these milks if your baby has significant and frequent vomiting, the premise being that the thickened milk can more easily stay in the stomach and not be refluxed out. These milks may reduce vomiting but will not affect pain caused from an acid-irritated oesophagus.

Anti-reflux milks designed to stop the posseting of reflux babies may not address other digestive difficulties.

Rice-thickened milks have been shown to increase risk of constipation in 36% of infants[83].

Milk thickened with carob bean gum is less nutritive because of the decreased bioavailability of essential nutrients. Two pre-term infants developed fatal necrotising enterocolitis after being given carob-bean-gum-thickened milks to reduce reflux regurgitation[84]. Further research and investigation is required, so for the moment carob-bean-gum-thickened milks should not be used for pre-term infants with this risk. In addition, observations made in the *Journal of Paediatrics* in 2015 mention a "possible association between necrotizing enterocolitis and ingestion of a commercial feed thickener by premature infants."[85]

Thickening agents themselves may cause problems for babies' digestion. Many are thickened with rice, which naturally contains arsenic. There are no safe limits for arsenic levels in infant diets, because of the immaturity of their bodies. The risks associated with arsenic consumption can lead to

---

83 https://www.ncbi.nlm.nih.gov/pubmed/16211190
84 Clarke, P, and M Robinson. "Thickening Milk Feeds May Cause Necrotising Enterocolitis." Archives of Disease in Childhood Fetal and Neonatal Edition 89.3 (2004): F280. PMC. Web. 28 Sept. 2017.
85 https://www.ncbi.nlm.nih.gov/pubmed/22575248

lower IQ, impaired brain development, growth problems, breathing problems, cancer as an adult and an impaired immune system[86].

Thickening with potato starch may reduce regurgitation, but may have a negative impact on the intestines causing greater bloating, abdominal pain, trapped wind and/or flatulence. This is because baby does not have the enzymes required to break down potato starch, so it can ferment when it reaches the gut.

6.1.3 Hypoallergenic (HA)/Partially Hydrolysed Formula

These milks have been treated so that the proteins in them have been broken down to make digestion easier for baby. They are not suitable for babies with cow's milk protein allergy and may not be suitable for lactose-intolerant babies either.

6.1.4 Extensively Hydrolysed Formula (EHF)

This milk has been treated with enzymes to break down most of the proteins that cause allergy symptoms, although the milk is still of cow origin. This is the usually the first recommended option for CMPA babies.

6.1.5 Amino-Acid-Based/Elemental Formula

These formulas are based on 100% non-allergenic amino acids that will not trigger an allergic reaction. Although these milks may not trigger confirmed IgE[87] response allergic reactions, baby can have an intolerance response to some of the ingredients.

In summary, you can see that no single milk provides a complete answer for any individual baby and it is important to remember this when trialling any new milk.

---

86 https://www.dartmouth.edu/~arsenicandyou/health/children.html

87 IgE is immunoglobulin-E, a specific antigen produced by the body in response to a positive immune system allergic response. It is immediate in its appearance in the body (within 2 hours). This is the most basic of "allergy" definitions. More information can be found in Section 9.

6.2   NUTRITIONAL MACROS OF INFANT FORMULA

6.2.1   PROTEIN CONTENT

Protein content of formula milks is another consideration to bear in mind. Mature human breastmilk is a delicately balanced and fine-tuned fluid that supports the needs of every individual baby. It is incredibly powerful in its dynamic ability to change its composition in response to what baby needs, not just on a macronutrient level, but on a micronutrient and immune system supportive level. Clearly, formula milk cannot adapt like this and does not respond to individual babies' needs.

Human milk is typically about 7% protein. All formula milks are more than 7% protein, some as high as 11% of energy from protein sources. A study published in the *American Journal of Clinical Nutrition* in 2014 concluded that childhood obesity risk for school-age children could be reduced by using lower protein content infant formula when compared with other formula milks[88]. The study did not include breastfed infants, and further research would be necessary to draw the conclusion that the lower protein content in breastmilk would reduce childhood obesity risk.

6.2.2   CARBOHYDRATE & FAT CONTENT

Human breastmilk is designed by nature to have the correct proportions of macronutrients to support babies' growth and development optimally. It provides between 53% and 55% of its energy from fat sources. Babies' digestive systems are designed to extract energy from fat efficiently. Of note, all baby formulas have less than 50% of energy provided from fat sources.

Fat is extremely important in the early development cycles of babies' brains, because brain tissue is built from fat cells. Fat is a vital macronutrient to support brain development and cognitive function. Higher fat milks would be preferable to higher carbohydrate milks.

---

88 http://ajcn.nutrition.org/content/early/2014/03/12/ajcn.113.064071.full.pdf+html

Human breastmilk has about 39% energy provided from carbohydrate sources, or sugars. Again, looking at the table of macronutrients, all formula milks are over 40% carbohydrate in terms of energy provision. This is important because not all of the formulas are readily digestible by baby, purely from the natural immaturity of their digestive systems.

6.3   FORMULA MILK CONTENTS: AN OVERVIEW

This section outlines many of the main tins of formula milk available for infants in the UK as at October 2017. Included here are the macros for each milk, as this is important considering the impact of high-protein formulas on infant growth.

As a baseline comparison, breastmilk changes dynamically in response to baby's needs, and so the proportions of protein, carbohydrate and fat can vary. It may contain allergens and indigestible elements depending on mother's diet; it is the most flexible and controllable because diet has a direct impact on "ingredients".

The table overleaf details the proportions of protein, carbohydrate and fat per 100ml of each milk in grams, and as a percentage of calorific energy provided by each macronutrient. The last column identifies those ingredients in the milk that are either likely allergens, or may present a digestive irritation due to the complexity of their structure.

Ingredients in *italics* indicate *potential allergens*, and **bold** indicate **indigestible ingredients** for infants that may ferment, causing gas, bloating and abdominal pain.

Milk	Protein per 100ml % of energy	Carbs per 100ml % of energy	Fat per 100ml % of energy	Ingredients that may cause irritation to a sensitive digestive system
Mature human milk[89]	1.3g 7%	7.0g 39%	4.2g 54%	See above
Cow's milk	3.2g 21%	4.8g 31%	3.3g 48%	Cow's milk
Neocate LCP[90]	1.8g 11%	7.2g 43%	3.4g 46%	Coconut oil
Similac Sensitive[91]	2.1g 8%	11.1 44%	5.4g 48%	Milk protein isolate, sugar, soy oil
Aptamil Comfort[92]	1.5g 6%	7.2g 44%	3.4g 47%	Hydrolysed whey protein concentrate (from milk), starch (potato, maize), galacto-oligosaccharides (GOS) (from milk), lactose (from milk), emulsifier (soy lecithin)
Aptamil Pepti 1[93]	1.6g 10%	7.0g 42%	3.5g 47%	Hydrolysed whey protein concentrate (from milk), maltodextrin, GOS (from milk), FOS, fish oil
Aptamil Pepti 2[94]	1.6g 10%	8.1g 49%	3.1g 42%	Maltodextrin, hydrolysed whey protein concentrate (from milk), GOS (from milk), FOS, fish oil
Aptamil Anti-Reflux[95]	1.6g 10%	6.8g 42%	3.5g 48%	Lactose (from milk), skimmed milk, maltodextrin, carob bean gum, fish oil, emulsifier (soy lecithin)

89 http://www.infantnutritioncouncil.com/resources/breastmilk-information/
90 http://www.neocate.co.uk/uploadedFiles/
Neocate/Resources_Library/Documents/Neocate_LCP_data_card.pdf
91 https://static.abbottnutrition.com/cms-prod/abbottnutrition-2016.com/img/Similac-Sensitive.pdf
92 https://eln.nutricia.co.uk/media/4352/datacard_aptamil_comfort.pdf
93 https://eln.nutricia.co.uk/media/4353/datacard_aptamil_pepti_1.pdf
94 https://eln.nutricia.co.uk/media/4355/datacard_aptamil_pepti_2.pdf
95 https://eln.nutricia.co.uk/media/4356/datacard_aptamil_anti_reflux.pdf

Milk	Protein per 100ml % of energy	Carbs per 100ml % of energy	Fat per 100ml % of energy	Ingredients that may cause irritation to a sensitive digestive system
Aptamil Lactose Free[96]	1.3g 8%	7.3g 44%	3.5g 48%	Caseinate (from milk), fish oil, emulsifier (soy lecithin)
Aptamil 1st Milk Powder[97]	1.3g 8%	7.3g 45%	3.4g 47%	Demineralised whey (from milk), lactose (from milk), skimmed milk, GOS (from milk), whey protein concentrate (from milk), FOS, fish oil, emulsifier (soy lecithin)
Aptamil Hungry Baby[98]	1.6g 10%	7.7g 47%	3.1g 43%	Lactose (from milk), skimmed milk, GOS (from milk), FOS, fish oil, emulsifier (soy lecithin)
Aptamil Profutura 1st Infant Formula[99]	1.3g 8%	7.0g 44%	3.4g 48%	Demineralised whey (from milk), lactose (from milk), skimmed milk, anhydrous milk fat, GOS (from milk), whey protein concentrate (from milk), Phospholipid (from egg), FOS, fish oil, emulsifier (soy lecithin)
Hipp Organic First Infant Milk 1[100]	1.25g 9%	7.3g 44%	3.5g 47%	Organic skimmed milk, organic whey powder, organic lactose, GOS from lactose, whey protein, fish oil, inositol
Hipp Organic Hungry Infant Milk[95]	1.6g 9%	7.3g 44%	3.5g 47%	Organic skimmed milk, organic lactose, GOS from lactose, fish oil
Hipp Organic Anti-Reflux Milk[95]	1.4g 9%	7.1g 43%	3.5g 48%	Organic skimmed milk, organic whey product, organic maltodextrin, carob bean gum, organic lactose, fish oil

96 https://eln.nutricia.co.uk/media/4354/datacard_aptamil_lactose_free.pdf
97 https://eln.nutricia.co.uk/media/4338/datacard_aptamil_first_milk.pdf
98 https://eln.nutricia.co.uk/media/4359/datacard_aptamil_hungry_milk.pdf
99 https://eln.nutricia.co.uk/media/4349/datacard_aptamil_profutura_first.pdf
100 https://www.hipp4hcps.co.uk/fileadmin/media_hcp/pdf/product_information_sheet_-_milks_range_ingredients_feb_2017.pdf

Milk	Protein per 100ml / % of energy	Carbs per 100ml / % of energy	Fat per 100ml / % of energy	Ingredients that may cause irritation to a sensitive digestive system
Hipp Combiotic Comfort Milk[95]	1.6g / 10%	7.1g / 43%	3.5g / 47%	Maltodextrin, lactose, whey protein hydrolysate, starch, GOS (from lactose), fish oil
Nanny Care Goat Milk Formula[101]	1.3g / 8%	7.4g / 45%	3.4g / 47%	Pasteurised goat milk solids (43%), lactose from milk (cow's milk)
Nutramigen Puramino[102]	1.89g / 11%	7.0g / 41%	3.6g / 48%	Corn syrup solids, Soy oil, modified tapioca starch
Similac Ailmentum[103]	1.9g / 11%	6.9g / 40%	3.7g / 49%	Corn maltodextrin, casein hydrolysate derived from milk, sugar, soy oil, xanthan gum
SMA PRO First Infant Milk[104]	1.25g / 8%	7.1g / 43%	3.6g / 49%	Lactose (from milk), demineralised whey (from milk), skimmed milk, emulsifier (soya lecithin), FOS, fish oil
SMA Hypoallergenic Infant Milk	1.3g / 8%	7.8g / 47%	3.4g / 46%	Lactose (from milk), partially hydrolysed whey protein (from milk), fish oil, inositol
Enfamil Infant[105]	2g / 8%	11.3g / 44%	12.3g / 48%	Non-fat milk, lactose, soy oil, whey protein concentrate, polydextrose, GOS, soy lecithin
Enfamil A.R.[106]	8%	44%	48%	Non-fat milk, rice starch, lactose, maltodextrin, polydextrose, soy oil

101 https://static1.squarespace.com/static/53f098cee4b0cc6081ee3265/t/
5425caece4b098d4a87a7666/1411762924219/NANNYcare_compositional+info3_4.pdf
102 https://www.meadjohnson.com/pediatrics/us-en/product-
information/products/infants/puramino#preparation-of-feedings
103 https://similac.com/baby-formula/similac-expert-care-alimentum
104 https://www.smababy.co.uk/formula-milk/first-infant-milk/
105 https://www.meadjohnson.com/pediatrics/us-en/product-information/products/infants/enfamil-
infant#product-characteristics
106 https://www.meadjohnson.com/pediatrics/us-en/product-information/products/infants/enfamil-a-r

Goat's formula milk may be an option for some babies with reflux because its fat globules are smaller than those of cow's milk, and so may support digestion in a gentler way. Goat's milk products are not suitable for babies with cow's milk sensitives to either casein (protein) or lactose (sugar).

Typically, the "hungry baby" milks contain more casein (milk protein) than whey, which is harder to digest. There is no evidence that it helps baby sleep longer or better[107].

Most formula milks contain galacto-oligosaccharides (GOS), which are prebiotics. These are non-digestible ingredients that support the growth and activity of the good bacteria in the gut. Fructo-oligosaccharides (FOS) are prebiotics too. They have a sweet taste so are often used as an artificial sweetener in products. FOS have been found to support calcium absorption. However, FOS are also fermented by pathogenic bacteria in the gut such as *Klebsiella*, *E. coli* and *Clostridium*, all of which are responsible for gas formation. These could pose a problem to babies suffering with painful wind and bloated tummies.

Note: The ready-to-drink formulas often have additional ingredients added over and above those for powdered milk. I have not assessed these formulas.

In January 2004, Sir Liam Donaldson, UK Chief Medical Officer, re-stated advice that "soya-based infant formulas should not be used as the first choice for the management of infants with proven cow's milk sensitivity, lactose intolerance, galactokinase deficiency and galactosaemia."[108] Earlier, in 2003, the Committee on Toxicity had already

---

107 http://www.nhs.uk/Conditions/pregnancy-and-baby/Pages/types-of-infant-formula.aspx

108 UK Department of Health. CMO's Update 37: Advice issued on soya-based infant formulas. 2004. http://webarchive.nationalarchives.gov.uk/20120503095605/http://www.dh.gov.uk/en/Publicationsandstatisti cs/Lettersandcirculars/CMOupdate/DH_4070172

stated that "soya-based formulas have a high phytoestrogen content, which could pose a risk to the long-term reproductive health of infants".

Note: Soya and soy are the same thing. This is US and UK nomenclature.

6.3.1   WHICH MILK?

Unless your baby is showing strong signs of allergy or intolerance, I suggest trying milks in the order outlined below. This is my personal opinion, based on the ingredients information for each product. Every baby is different, and so there is no one-size-fits-all solution.

I start with the milks with fewest complex sugars to minimise fermentation in baby's gut; baby should be able to digest them more easily. This list gradually moves from gentle and easier-to-digest milks; move through them one at a time if symptoms continue to be observed after 5 days.

So that you have a written record of what is going on, I recommend keeping a milk and symptom diary. Try a milk for at least 5 days (unless there is a dramatic and clear allergy reaction such as rash or difficulty breathing); in which case, you should stop the particular milk completely and return to the previous best milk.

Once you have found a milk that works for your baby, stop there and keep feeding that milk.

1. Hipp Organic 1st Milk
2. Nanny Care Goat Milk Formula
3. Aptamil Lactose Free
4. SMA Hypoallergenic Infant Milk
5. Neocate LCP

7   ALL YOU NEED TO KNOW ABOUT FOOD

Using food to manage intolerances in your baby can be hugely beneficial for a breastfeeding mum as well as for the child. You may not realise it but foods that impact your baby may also be having an impact on your body, perhaps to a lesser degree than your child, but you can still have massive benefits by changing what you eat. You'll see this as a bonus benefit alongside improvements to your child's comfort and health.

Some of the benefits you may achieve (just like I did!) include:

- Weight loss – over the first month of my elimination diet, I lost 14 lbs (1 stone), weight I had assumed was just stuck on me, as I thought I had already lost my baby weight.

- Clearer mind, improved concentration – the new way of eating allowed my brain to stop being clouded, massively reducing 'baby brain' even though my sleep didn't improve for a while.

- Better moods – I experienced way fewer mood swings as my sugar intake reduced to virtually zero.

- Willpower increase – I found that when I was doing something for the good of my child's health, it was far easier to stick to it than for my own health. Also, it directly impacted sleep on the same night, so I had a clear incentive to stick to the foods I knew were fine for both of us.

7.1   INTOLERANCES & ALLERGIES

It is especially difficult to diagnose an allergy or intolerance, or to tell them apart one from the other. Symptoms can be virtually identical in many cases and the variety of symptoms observable is huge.

From a physiological perspective, there is a way to tell the difference, and that is a skin-prick test or radioallergosorbent (RAST) test done by blood testing that checks for IgE specific antigens in the blood indicating an immune system response. An alternative is identifying the problem substance through a food diary.

From a treatment perspective, there is little difference in what happens next: a process of constructing menus and arranging your life so that you avoid the culprit(s) interfering with your day-to-day.

If your child has an allergic response that is at anaphylaxis level, evidently there is no sense in risking life. Identify the allergen(s) with the help of a professional immunologist or allergist, and remove the allergen from your home entirely. For example, if your child has a strong allergy to dairy, I suggest not having milk, butter, cheese etc in your home for any occasion, not even if you have guests. They will understand that you are putting the life of your child first.

If the skin-prink test comes back positive for an allergy, then your baby is allergic to that food/substance and it should be avoided. However, if the test is negative, it is *not conclusive* that your baby is not allergic to those allergens. The only way of knowing for certain is elimination and re-introduction with keen observation.

The following table outlines the differences and commonalities between allergies and intolerances.

Characteristic	Allergy	Intolerance
Time lag to symptom showing up	Immediate: Seconds after exposure to 2 hours	Medium to short term, usually a few hours up to 4 days
Symptoms	Anaphylaxis Difficulty breathing Dizziness Loss of Consciousness	Never anaphylaxis
	Skin Hives Itchiness Swelling Rash Eczema Psoriasis	Skin Hives Itchiness Swelling Rash Eczema Psoriasis
	Gastrointestinal Vomiting Diarrhoea	Gastrointestinal Vomiting Diarrhoea Abdominal pain Bloating Gas Trapped wind
	Respiratory, usually don't occur alone Difficulty breathing Runny nose Sneezing Wheezing Coughing Asthma	Respiratory, usually don't occur alone Difficulty breathing Runny nose Sneezing Wheezing Coughing Asthma
Severity	Can be fatal if not treated immediately and properly	Can cause discomfort and pain but rarely life-threatening
Body system affected	Immune system – production of antibodies called Immunoglobulin-E (IgE).	Digestive system with knock-on effects of symptoms sometimes showing up elsewhere (e.g. skin, respiratory). May show up as IgG (delayed response)

Management	Severe allergies where there is a potential risk of anaphylaxis will have an EpiPen prescribed by the doctor.	General awareness and avoidance of irritants
	Anyone caring for your child must be properly trained (for example, in the use of an EpiPen)	Putting up with the symptoms until they have passed through the body is all that can be done
	Extreme caution and care should be taken to avoid the allergen at all costs	
	With minor allergic reactions, ongoing awareness	Active management to support the elimination of the irritant from the body (e.g. tummy massage, reflexology, herbal teas)
	Antihistamines may help calm symptoms quickly and effectively (this must be under the guidance of your GP)	
	Often allergy symptoms are treated with steroids rather than identifying and avoiding the allergen. This, however, brings its own risks[109]:	
	Reduced growth in children	
	Increased risk of infection due to a less effective immune system	
	Weight gain	
	Fluid retention	
	Moon-shaped face	
	Skin problems	
	Hardening of the arteries (which can lead to heart disease)	
	Increased blood sugar levels (which can contribute to diabetes)	
	Mood swings	
	Insomnia	
	Other gastrointestinal problems	
	Thinning of bones	
	Eye problems	
	Cushing's syndrome	

In relation to allergies in any babies, Allergy UK includes reflux as a delayed symptom of a food allergy[110]. This reference also defines the following list as symptoms of delayed food allergies:

---

109 https://www.webmd.boots.com/a-to-z-guides/side-effects-long-term-steroid-use
110 https://www.allergyuk.org/information-and-advice/conditions-and-symptoms/42-childhood-food-allergy

- Eczema
- Reflux – an effortless vomiting
- Poor growth
- Swelling in the small bowel
- Constipation and/or diarrhoea
- Raising knees to chest with tummy pain
- Frequent distress and crying

Wouldn't it be amazing if we could determine which foods were likely to cause an allergic reaction or intolerance response from our baby before we introduce the food? The unfortunate fact is the only true way to test a food is to consume it.

Having said that, if a baby's parents have known food allergies, there is a slightly increased risk that baby will be allergic to that same foodstuff. However, the risk is low, so there is no reason to avoid foods where a parent has an allergy. Rather, you should have more observation around these foods when being introduced.

7.1.1   ORAL FOOD CHALLENGE

The gold standard for diagnosis is an oral food challenge. This is consuming the suspected food in gradually increasing amounts combined with careful observation to see if *any* symptoms arise. Not, as I have observed in some cases, keep consuming it until the symptoms are unbearable.

If no symptoms consistent with an IgE allergy occur (hives, swelling, anaphylaxis), then it can be said that an IgE allergy response to that food is unlikely. The period of observation for this response is up to 8 hours. If no symptoms occur within 4 days of the food consumption, then there is no intolerance to that food and it is safe for baby to have.

If your child has a known allergy, then the oral challenge must be done under the clinical supervision of your allergist in the proper setting as deemed by them. Your greatest assets in understanding an oral challenge are:

- Starting from a place of "good", ideally symptom-free
- Using a food and symptom diary
- Observations (either yourself or people around your child)

7.1.2   PATCH-TESTING

This is most effective if your baby has any skin conditions or symptoms such as eczema or dermatitis. However, because this is so easy to do, it can be useful as a basic indicator for new potential allergen foods.

Skin patch tests will show results for non-IgE response (delayed IgG/intolerance) foods. Skin patch tests do not pick up every intolerance, but those that they do detect are definite substances to avoid.

In particular, I recommend these tests for the bathing and baby care products that you're using with your child, including:

- Wipes
- Shampoo
- Bath additives (bubble mixtures, skin softeners, moisturisers e.g. Oilatum etc)
- Baby creams
- Foods

Exclude known allergens to your baby from patch tests.

A patch test is simple to do and overnight is easiest. Before you start, make sure your baby is in good health with no compromised breathing such as congestion, snoring or coughing.

1. Get a small piece of the food/substance to be tested
2. Mix it with a little water
3. Using a cotton bud, rub a little of the paste on the inside of your baby's wrist. This is most easily done just after baby has fallen asleep as they are less likely to wipe it off before it dries.
4. If you notice an immediate reaction, wipe the area clean with some cotton wool and water immediately. This is an allergen.

5. Check for reactions after 15 minutes, after 1 hour and then before you go to bed. If you notice any reaction, wipe the area clean.
6. In the morning, check the area to see if there has been any reaction. A reaction can show up as a welt, redness, rash or hives.

Pay close attention to baby and check they are sleeping normally. If you see any noticeable chances, phone 101 (in the UK), your out-of-hours GP, or emergency response as you believe to be best.

Keep a record of what foods and substances you test, when and what reactions occur.

7.2   MINIMISING ALLERGEN RESPONSE

A relative lack of early microbial exposure (including gastrointestinal and respiratory) can contribute to babies developing allergic reactions and diseases. A logical way to reduce allergic sensitivity, therefore, is to support and build up baby's own microbiome as early as possible. There are several ways in which you can achieve this:

1. Natural birth – before baby is born, their gut has a lower density of bacteria and a culture reflective of oral bacteria. The passage through the vaginal canal naturally exposes them to microbes and boosts the population of their gut and intestinal flora, or microbiome.
2. Skin-to-skin contact – once born and in early life, the baby will increase exposure to "normal" bacteria strengthening the microbiome.
3. Breastfeeding – breastmilk promotes the colonisation and maturation of the infant gut microbiome due to the bacteria contained within it. Breastmilk also contains sugars specific to promoting the growth of beneficial microbial communities, because not all gut bacteria have been created equal!
4. Supplementation for baby – a combined prebiotic and probiotic for baby, so as to support growth and development of a healthy

and productive gut microbiome[111]. Take care in selecting a prebiotic and probiotic as many contain strains derived from dairy sources, which can irritate a baby's immature digestive system.

5. Supplementation for breastfeeding mums – a good probiotic for breastfeeding mothers. Probiotics support the strong growth of mothers' gut flora, which influences the bacteria present in the breastmilk.

7.3   REFLUX FLARES WITH SOLIDS

The standard Western diet that we are advised to give our babies from 6 months of age is designed to fit in "culturally" with us and our babies, but apparently also for convenience. We tend to think whatever is mass-produced and readily available should be fed to baby; this is not necessarily the case.

The approach in this book focusses on what is *best for baby*. And only what is best for baby. I don't mess around pretending that babies are or should be able to eat an adult diet from the age of 6 months. I respect their still-developing digestive systems and look at what they can digest as well as the nutritional value and benefit from meals.

I can see where the phrase "food before 1 is just for fun" comes in. Too many mums think their baby should be eating three wholesome and filling meals per day at 6 months, or even progressing from no solids to three meals per day by 9 months with an infinitely variable diet.

This belief puts too much pressure on mums and babies. Mums feel the need to be like a chef in a restaurant, afraid of not giving baby a varied diet both in colour, shape, size and the funniest faces on a plate. Babies will feel it on the digestive system, with too much change too quickly.

---

111 https://www.ncbi.nlm.nih.gov/pmc/articles/PMC4464665/

The truth is baby needs to *learn* how to eat. Their digestive system needs to adjust to a new diet and not suddenly jump to three meals per day. The transition should look like a gradual build-up to food and a conscious introduction of food so that baby's digestive system is not over-stressed.

Many babies experience a flare-up of reflux symptoms when they start on solids. Regardless of medication, it can feel like things are as bad as ever, maybe even worse.

There is hope.

I have a food introduction programme I have designed specifically around the development of an infants' digestive ability, so that food supports baby, with minimal reflux flares and quick identification if one should. And I teach parents how to safely and gradually grow the diet to a very varied, healthy diet.

PART 3

FOOD FOR
REFLUX BABIES

8   FOOD FOR BABIES

The standard food pyramid from the 1980s is what most people know and use to influence their daily food choices. This is a carbohydrate-loaded system and is not suitable for a baby's growth and development. Instead, the World Health Organization (WHO) recommends that babies should be breastfed until the age of 2 for optimal development. "WHO recommends mothers worldwide to exclusively breastfeed infants for the child's first 6 months to achieve optimal growth, development and health. Thereafter, they should be given nutritious complementary foods and continue breastfeeding up to the age of 2 years or beyond."[112]

The recommendations do not include giving children cow's milk at 1 year, nor formula milk. WHO makes a specific recommendation about continuing breastmilk until the age of 2. The benefits for children who have had breastmilk until 2 years of age compared to those who stopped at 6 months include:

- providing up to half or more of a child's nutritional needs during the second half of the first year, and up to one-third during the second year of life
- promoting sensory and cognitive development
- protecting the infant against infectious and chronic diseases
- reducing infant mortality due to common childhood illnesses such as diarrhoea or pneumonia, and quicker recovery during illness

Furthermore, breastfeeding contributes to the health and wellbeing of mothers, helps to space children, reduces the risk of ovarian cancer and

---

112 WHO Statement ,15 January 2011,
http://www.who.int/mediacentre/news/statements/2011/breastfeeding_20110115/en/

breast cancer, increases family and national resources, is a secure way of feeding and is safe for the environment.

The WHO advises that first foods for babies are often the staple (carbohydrate) food of the community; for example, porridge, bread, rice etc. I strongly disagree that such starchy carbohydrates should be first foods for babies with sensitive digestive systems after my learning of how baby's digestive system develops.

"The basic ingredient of complementary foods is usually the local staple. Staples are cereals, roots and starchy fruits that consist mainly of carbohydrate and provide energy."[113]

On no account do I believe there is any excuse for compromising the comfort or health of any baby on the basis that food is "the starch of the community" or is "cheap"; these types of food can be more irritating to the immature digestive system rather than supportive and gentle. Sure, I understand the need for parents to be able to afford to feed their children, but over a period of 12-60 months, I suggest the cost of food averages out for several reasons:

- children given foods of higher nutritional and energy density will snack less
- children given higher nutritional foods will require less volume of food
- they will be healthier, requiring fewer doctor visits or prescription medicines

If better food principles were to be adopted on a large scale basis, it could impact the health of the child and indeed the nation. Instead of

---

113 Infant and Young Child Feeding: Model Chapter for Textbooks for Medical Students and Allied Health Professionals. Geneva: World Health Organization; 2009. Available from: https://www.ncbi.nlm.nih.gov/books/NBK148965/

subsidising medications, government could and should be subsidising proper food for infants and children.

8.1   Baby Food, The Aine Way

8.1.1   Basis of Infant Macronutritional Requirements

After 4 years of experimenting, reading, researching, food diaries and food management, I have developed my own theories about the food I am willing to feed my children. I have several "rules" that I apply to daily life and a set of guidelines about how to "break the rules" and when.

I love the phrase that the WHO uses for introducing foods to infants – *complementary* feeding. The food should complement baby's milk; it is not a replacement; together with milk, it is *part* of baby's nourishment.

Since breastmilk is *designed* for infants, I believe any complementary or replacement foods should reflect the changing nutritional qualities of breastmilk up to 3 years of age, and be the required fuel for infant, baby and toddler development. Food for babies ought to have the energy and nutrients that they require.

The first 2 years of life is the fastest period of growth they will experience across all areas – physical growth, motor development, brain growth and development, emotional wellbeing and understanding who they are as a person. The most important part of this development, in my opinion, is the brain. If optimal fuel for brain development – emotional, mechanical, creative, physical, communicative, cognitive – is available to the body, the overall development of the infant and child will be accelerated.

I don't mean that the child "grows up quicker", but rather learning becomes effortless, behavioural skills develop without stress and the child will tend to be less upset over some happenings in their life.

In short, I advocate that complementary food should be high in *good* fat, moderate in protein and moderate in *simple* carbohydrates. The child's diet should avoid most processed foods and be free of refined sugar and wheat[114].

8.1.2   THE MIND-SHIFT

There is a mind-shift needed when feeding babies. Your baby's digestive system is designed to maximise energy from fat. Their body produces a higher number of fat-digesting enzymes than an adult. They should be getting 55% of their calorie intake from fat sources, about 39% from carbohydrates and 6% from protein sources. This is the representative calorific value of breastmilk.

It is not necessary for your baby to be having substantial carbohydrates at a young age. I advise all my clients to stay away from breads and pastas as these are complex carbohydrates that baby simply does not have the appropriate enzymes to digest effectively until they have all their milk teeth.

When it comes to introducing solids, we need to remove our own personal preconceptions from the equation. We need to stop projecting our feelings and beliefs onto our babies, and allow our babies the opportunity to experience food without the internal conversations that *we* have going on.

"Fats are bad for me…
I must stay away from white food…
I hate broccoli, or anything that is green…
Furry fruit is 'wrong'…
I need carbs to feel full…
Dinner isn't a meal without a spud…"

That last one is for the Irish out there, but has a serious note to us all.

---

114 If feeding wheat to a child, I suggest only an ancient variety (e.g. Einkorn) and sprouted or fermented grains as in a high quality sourdough bread.

We must step away from how our own bodies react to and feel about food, and instead support our babies the way they need. We must realise that from a basic physiological level, our babies' bodies are not the same as ours. They cannot digest food in the same way. And this is *normal*.

Your baby does not need "bulk" like adults typically do. Your baby needs energy and nutrition from food. Therefore, baby food should offer energy and nutrition as its primary focus, not the feeling of "being full up".

Your baby uses their instinct, their "gut feeling", a lot more than an adult, and we should trust our babies' choices of food. We must understand that how our babies perceive and experience food in their own bodies is massively important for how they will be able to trust in it, listen to what it is telling them, and choose the right food and nourishment for themselves. There are, of course, some exceptions, but generally I believe our babies naturally choose what is best for them, given the correct support.

The work of Clara Marie Davis on child self-selection of (healthy) foods, where a number of children (followed for up to 4½ years) were offered a range of healthy foods and were allowed to freely choose and eat whatever they wanted, in whatever quantity, resulted in all 15 participants growing into "uniformly well-nourished, healthy children."[115] Her work was also approved and promoted by Dr Benjamin Spock. He wrote that a mother "can trust an unspoiled child's appetite to choose a wholesome diet if she serves him a reasonable variety and balance of those natural and unrefined foods *which he himself enjoys eating at present* [Dr. Spock's emphasis] [...] Even more importantly, it means that she doesn't have to worry when he develops a temporary dislike of a vegetable."[116]

No single meal or even day of food needs to be perfectly balanced. With young babies, and indeed with older children, we are seeking to

---

115 Strauss S. Clara M. Davis and the wisdom of letting children choose their own diets. CMAJ : Canadian Medical Association Journal. 2006;175(10):1199-1201. doi:10.1503/cmaj.060990.

116 Spock B. The common sense book of baby and child care. New York: Duell, Sloan and Pearce; 1946. p. 527.

balance their overall diet. Looking at this from a weekly point of view is rather pleasing. You may find days when you baby only wants to eat fruit. Another day meat. Another day just overloads on broccoli! This is okay. Look at the week as a whole.

The mind-shift is tricky, especially as your support group may not understand what you are thinking. That's why I've written this book – to provide all the information you need to do this.

8.2   BALANCING NUTRITION & CALORIES

At 6 months, baby's digestive system is still designed to digest milk and to get their energy requirements from that milk. To minimise the stress introduced to the body when baby starts eating and to learn as effectively as possible, I believe baby's energy intake should mimic the balance they have in milk.

As I mentioned above, in milk, 55% of the calories (energy) come from fat, 39% from carbohydrates and 6% from protein. All of these macronutrients are in the simplest form available to the digestive system.

As they grow, babies need more calories, based on their weight. The table overleaf shows the approximate daily calorie requirements per pound and kilogram of weight of your baby. From this, you can easily calculate how much "energy" your child should be consuming[117].

Age	kCal/lb/day	kCal/kg/day
0 – 6 months	50-55*	110-120*
6 – 12 months	45*	95-100*
15 years	20	44

117   http://www.msdmanuals.com/en-gb/professional/pediatrics/care-of-newborns-and-infants/nutrition-in-infants#v1076566

*When protein and calories are provided by breastmilk that is completely digested and absorbed, the requirements between 3 and 9 months of age may be lower.

Weight	**kCal/kg/day**
11 lbs/5 kg	475-500 kCal
13.2 lbs/6 kg	570–600 kCal
18 lbs/8.2kg	780-820 kCal
19 lbs/8.6 kg	820–860 kCal
20 lbs/9.0 kg	855–900 kCal
21 lbs/9.5 kg	900–950 kCal
22 lbs/10 kg	950–1,000 kCal

Remember, the aim is not for baby to get all of these calories from food as they will still be drinking significant amounts of milk.

Recalling the proportions of calories from fat, carbohydrates and protein, obviously, it would be tricky to mimic the 55:39:6 ratio perfectly or in every meal. Rather I am suggesting that infant feeding should move away from loading baby with carbs (the disaccharides they can't digest) at 6 months and focussing on nutritionally dense food rather than volume.

Nutritional density is the amount of valuable nutrition crammed into a particular volume of food. It describes how much nutrition (including energy) we can get from the same mass of different foods. For example, an egg is more nutritious per 100g than bread, but wholemeal bread is more nutritionally dense than white bread as there are more macro and micronutrients in the wholemeal version.

In the Western world, adults have become accustomed to eating carbs as our primary source of energy. Yet this has led us to being a generally unhealthy society, when the carbs we eat are lacking in nutritional content. I would like to see our infants shifting to a healthier way of eating that teaches them and their bodies much more about nutrition and feeling healthy early in life, rather than being in the high-risk category for obesity.

It's a real concern when 20% of children in the UK are obese by the age of 5[118].

8.3   THE MACROS

The three primary or macronutrients that we are all aware of are fats, proteins and carbohydrates. I add fluids as a forth and most important macro for babies, especially as they consume a 100% fluid diet for the first few months of life. I want to outline why and how these are important to our babies' development, and give you good sources of these nutrients.

8.3.1   FLUIDS

Fluid intake is so important in babies, because dehydration can occur quickly. Assess fluids daily, as a minimum. There are aspects that affect the fluid intake required by your baby, including milk type, fibre in the diet etc.

When your baby is drinking milk as their only source of nutrition, you are advised not to feed water as well. I understand the reason for this is that we want to make sure that baby is getting adequate nutrition from their fluid intake and additional water may reduce the volume of milk. However, water is not devoid of nutrition itself, often containing key minerals and salts dissolved within it. Additionally, depending on which milk your baby is drinking, water could play a part in supporting their growth and development.

Breastfed babies do not need additional water. However, if your baby is drinking a thickened formula or anti-reflux milk, which often results in constipation, the constipation itself is a signal that the milk is removing too much water from the baby's system. Baby needs more water, not more milk, in that case. More milk will just worsen the problem.

Understanding thickened milk, the reason a thickener is added is so that it reduces the free liquid in the drink. But doing this does not just thicken

---

118 http://www.rcpch.ac.uk/system/files/protected/page/SOCH-early-years-UK-2017.pdf

the milk. When the formula is consumed, it continues to absorb fluid from the gut, thereby reducing the amount of fluid available for your baby's body to function properly. Constipation and dry hard stools are classic signals that there is insufficient fluid in baby's body.

8.3.2   FATS

High quality fats are the most important part of baby's development. They are the easiest to digest, the basis for brain growth, critical to produce hormones that stimulate and control growth and development, and highest in energy density of all the macro food groups. Contrary to belief, good quality fats do not make people – babies, children, teenagers, or adults – fat. Your baby has an enhanced ability to digest fat because they produce lipase (a primary enzyme for the breakdown of fat) in the stomach, more so than an adult, while their pancreas continues to mature fully.

Fats are the foundational building blocks for brain tissue. Lightbulb! Yes, in the first 2 years of life, your baby's brain is growing and developing at a rate faster than it will ever do again. Their little body is designed to digest fat, the primary source for the building blocks of their brain, the organ that will then control everything else, from how they learn to how they grow, how they climb to how they throw.

Importantly, fats do not ferment in the body like carbs and proteins can, and so they do not cause the same bloating, gas and abdominal discomfort that we often observe from complex carbs in reflux babies.

The esteemed Harvard professor for child health and development, Jack P. Shonkoff M.D. is frequently quoted as saying, "Brains are built not born". Surely we should be ensuring that our babies have the best building blocks for their brain development that we can provide.

FASCINATING FAT FACTS

Fats are a vital structural part of every single cell in the body, regardless of the cell's function.

Fats are needed for the body to digest and absorb fat-soluble vitamins – A, D, E and K.

Fats support the digestion and use of protein in the body.

Fats are a fabulous source of energy.

Fats do not trigger insulin, and so do not trigger the sugar spike issue we experience with sugar and carbs.

Fats trigger the satiation mechanism – the release of dopamine from the brain, which in turn stops us from over-consuming. Fats make the body feel fuller sooner and for longer.

Fats are the building blocks of all hormones, which control every bodily function.

DIETARY SOURCES OF GOOD FAT

Fats are found all over nature, sometimes even in places we don't think to look. Make sure that your baby is eating adequate supplies of fat from these amazing sources:

- Egg yolks
- Avocado
- Coconut and coconut oil, milk and cream
- Cocoa butter (in dark chocolate or used as an ingredient itself)
- Cream (cow and goat)
- Cheeses (cow, sheep and goat)
- Animal fats – lard, tallow, bacon drippings, goose and duck fat
- Untreated vegetable oils – olive, avocado, nut
- Nuts (smooth nut butters and ground nuts, not whole or chopped nuts)
- Oily fish (e.g. salmon, trout, mackerel, herring, sardines)
- Meat (especially minced/ground meat with 20% fat), duck, goose
- Chia seeds
- Flax seed (freshly ground)
- Full-fat yogurt (cow and goat, or coconut)
- Butter (cow and goat)

- Mayonnaise (homemade from the fabulous ingredients above)
- Olives
- Meat (beef, pork, lamb)
- Poultry (Duck, goose)

INCLUDING FAT IN YOUR BABY'S DIET

Foods such as avocados, egg yolks, meats, cheese and yogurts can form quite a large part of any meal for your child. Ground nuts can be used in baked goods such as muffins, oils can be used in place of dips and sauces, butter and oils can be added to vegetables, and seeds and ground nuts can be made into puddings. There are infinite ways to combine foods for your baby.

Per gram, fats provide over twice the amount of energy than either protein or carbohydrates. If you have a picky eater, or a baby who likes small portions, or you want to up the calorie consumption of your baby for various reasons, then fats are the best choice.

TAKING CARE OF YOUR FATS

What is most important is that you look after the fats that are not in their natural state, specifically vegetable oils. Many fat extraction processes damage fats, meaning they are more bad than good by the time they reach our supermarkets. As such, there are some fats that you should never cook with – flax oil being one – because even low heat can damage them.

Light damages vegetable oils too. When purchasing your oil, buy one that is in an opaque bottle or an undamaged can. The less light the oil has been exposed to, the safer it is to consume.

Store your fats in a dark cupboard away from any heat sources such as your oven, hob, fridge, freezer or sun. This will keep them fresher longer, protect them from light and prevent them from going rancid. This maintains the safe goodness in them for your baby.

When cooking with fats, the lower the polyunsaturated content, the more stable the fat will be at high temperatures. Don't be afraid of cooking with animal fats like butter (grass-fed), lard, tallow (not for CMPA babies) goose and duck fat. Use them in cooking. The safest oil for cooking is coconut oil. If you want to avoid the "floral" tones added to everything by coconut oil, get the odourless (sans aroma) version; still a fabulous fat source, no taste is added to the food by the oil, so it enhances the flavour of what you are eating, and provides great nutrition and energy. In addition, coconut oil is an excellent source of medium chain triglycerides (MCTs) which require no digestion before being absorbed and used by our bodies as energy.

Animal fats, olive, avocado and nut oils are also good choices for stable cooking.

FATS TO AVOID

Contrary to popular belief, rapeseed oil (canola oil in the US) is a damaging oil and should not be consumed by infants. It undergoes extremely harsh processing that involves the use of a toxic solvent called hexane, among other chemicals. Bleach is also added to canola oil before bottling to lighten its colour.

All high-heat-treated oils – oils for deep frying – can be damaging. In small doses, our adult bodies can cope with this and detox ourselves. Older children are probably okay with small doses of these fats too. However, your baby does not need deep frying oils so please stay away from them. This includes any frozen products that have been deep fried in their preparation including all crisps.

8.3.3   CARBOHYDRATES

The group of food we all know and love. Or we *think* we know and we love, maybe love a little too much.

When we hear that babies need lots of energy, we might assume that we must provide high levels of carbohydrates. However, per gram, carbohydrates are the least efficient method of giving the body energy. In addition, they can be difficult to digest and have the lowest number of associated nutrients, vitamins and minerals.

A diet high in carbohydrates doesn't make sense for a young child who requires high levels of nutrition to support all areas of growth and development. Carbohydrates are necessary, don't get me wrong, but I do not believe that they should be the main part of every meal for a young child. In the case of breastfeeding children, heavy carbs don't need to feature at all among their foods.

Importantly, not all carbs are created equal. The carbs that babies need are those that also provide higher levels of specific minerals for growth and development. Babies do not need cereals that have been fortified with iron or any other mineral. They are much better off getting their mineral needs met from food sources – fruit, vegetables and animal products where the minerals are naturally occurring.

For years, we have been hearing from the nutritionist, dieticians and medics of the world that "white" foods are bad for us in general and we should stay away from them. You have been told that they cause blood sugar and insulin spikes. You have been told that they are low in nutritional value. Most of this is true. And yet, we're told to feed our babies white carbohydrates.

During the processing of "white" grains, the bran and germ are removed. Wheat, once ground, is often "fortified" with calcium, folic acid etc. A true, properly grown and unadulterated grain provides all the nutrition we require in the grain; it does not need to be fortified or improved. Fortification of a flour doesn't only add back in nutrients that were removed by the processing in the first place, but also provides additional bulk to the food substance, which essentially makes the true ingredient you are purchasing "go further" for the manufacturer. Typically, the quality of what is added back in is not in line with what was removed through processing. The calcium that is added is often not accessible to the human body – it has zero bioavailability and there is no point in feeding it to your baby.

All of this means wheat and sugar, as refined substances, are complete no-no's for an infant's diet. There is no health benefit for feeding either of these to your baby. Plus, both are complex carbohydrates that pose a fermentation problem to babies.

Potatoes should not be considered as a "bad food" because they are white in their natural state. They have not been through a refining process. They have considerable nutritional value and can be a healthy addition to meals at the appropriate age.

Are any carbs good for our babies then?

Carbohydrates are foods primarily made up of a number of sugar molecules, or "saccharides". Simple carbs are monosaccharides (one-sugar molecules) and complex carbs are disaccharides (two-sugar molecules), polysaccharides and oligosaccharides (multiple-sugar molecules).

Your baby can only break down and absorb simple sugars until their digestive system matures and they produce their own pancreatic amylase (around the time they have all their milk teeth). Until this point, baby only produces amylase (the enzyme for carbohydrate breakdown) in their saliva.

Disaccharides only get partially broken down or not at all. Polysaccharides and oligosaccharides are starches and fibre. Within the fibre group there are water soluble and insoluble fibres. Starches act like disaccharides. They may get partially broken down, but ultimately ferment and cause abdominal distress in the infant.

Water soluble fibres from grains absorb water from the digestive tract, causing constipation and inhibiting the intestines' ability to move nutrients into the blood.

Insoluble fibre is also known as cellulose, which is a plant structure not broken down by the body's enzymes. Importantly, it does not remove water from the body, but supports the movement of food in a gentle manner. These foods are often "prebiotics", which feed the good gut bacteria, and support positive microbiome development and growth.

Of these carbohydrates, babies should only eat monosaccharides and insoluble fibre. These foods allow your baby to digest what they are eating and get the nutrition from it. They support strong digestive system development.

EASILY DIGESTIBLE CARBS

Babies therefore need carbohydrates that are easily digested by their immature system. In the right form, carbs are perfectly okay for babies and children to consume in their natural state.

Monosaccharides do not rely on any enzymatic activity to be broken down further, and are ready to link with a transporter to cross the intestinal wall, and be absorbed and used by the body.

The most common monosaccharides are glucose (also known as dextrose), fructose and galactose. Foods high in monosaccharides include soft and tropical fruits[119]. As a treat, children can have natural fruit juices. The challenge with juices is that they have the fibre removed. In normal digestion of fruit, the fruit and the fibre are consumed at the same time and the body has to work through the fibre to release the sugars. The energy release from the food is naturally controlled, as it takes longer to breakdown. There is no sugar spike in this instance.

When fruit is consumed in juice or smoothie form, sugars are immediately available in the liquid. Whether or not the substance of the fruit is contained in the drink, like in a smoothie, the sugars from the fruit are available to be absorbed quickly into the bloodstream. The fibre in a smoothie has zero blood sugar regulation in-built. Therefore, this is almost like feeding baby a spoonful of sugar from the point of view of their blood sugar and insulin response.

---

119 Not all soft fruits are suitable for baby, so please continue to read this section before deciding on the foods you will select for you infant.

OTHER CONSIDERATIONS AROUND "SWEETS" AND SUGARS

Of course, babies should be allowed to experience sweet foods just as their taste buds are exposed to savoury. I believe this should be regulated and not overdone. Do not use food as a reward on a regular basis. Request that your family respects your choice. Do not reward children with sweets and chocolate. Yes, of course, you can have a special occasion, such as a birthday celebration, Christmas or Thanksgiving that involves additional special foods, but not just for good behaviour, as this will ultimately lead to ongoing poor behaviour. The link between behaviour and sugar is quickly observable.

The journey to knowing what to feed my children was by no means perfect. I made mistakes and learned from them. I'm learning all the time. My greatest tip is to continue observing.

I used to think that smoothies and pure fruit juices were acceptable for my girls. I used to also think that dried pureed fruit rolls were okay for my girls. Both were made from the fruit, the whole fruit and nothing but the fruit.

However, after a few weeks of letting my girls have a smoothie a day and a small packet of pure fruit chews, I started pulling my hair out about their behaviour in the afternoon. *Every* afternoon, without fail, they would be at each other's throats. And they were only 18 and 40 months! They fought and had to be separated. My eldest had tantrums and zero emotional control. She was only 3½ years old, but compared to her behaviour that same morning, when I could reason with her, this was like a different child. She would bite me, bite her little sister, scream and kick and throw toys around the house. She could not be pleased with anything.

One day, something clicked – it **had** to be the sugar in their diet. The next morning I told Sunflower and Daffodil that we were going to have an experiment and see if they could be nicer to each other all day. A sticker reward chart went up on the fridge. They had whole fruit, water and hot chocolate (my own recipe of almond milk and cocoa) at snack times.

I made sure they had proper meals. They asked – probably begged – for their smoothie and fruit rolls a few times, but I was so convinced in my theory that I found it easy to stick to my guns and say, "Sorry girls, we don't have any. It's that simple. I can't give you what I don't have in the house". No arguments.

The result was astounding.

That afternoon's behaviour was just like the morning. There was no biting. Any little fracas was just that – little and easily resolved. My patience was not tested. Sunflower and Daffodil were still best friends at bedtime and we had no real disruptive behaviour all day.

This became the new normal.

It doesn't mean they never had fruit smoothies or fruit rolls again. I reserve these for treats as a much healthier option to soft drinks and sweets. There is an understanding that sometimes they get treats, like mummy gets a coffee. Because this isn't a daily or weekly occurrence, they see it as a treat and like it as a treat. As a result, no behavioural issues! And importantly it is never given as a reward.

The other time I use fruit juice is when they are ill and I need to get fluids into them. Sunflower isn't always great at drinking water, so when I need her to increase her fluid intake, I will mix her water with some apple juice in a 2:1 water-juice ratio. I have found that diluting an apple or orange juice with two-thirds water reduces the chances of high blood sugar spikes that we see with undiluted fruit juice.

THE SCIENCE OF CARBOHYDRATES

The group of complex carbohydrates is more usefully broken down as sugars, starches and fibre. These are not strictly scientific definitions, yet they are sufficient in this context to understand how the molecular level differences in these sugars interact with the developing infantile digestive system.

Carbohydrates are built from monosaccharides as building blocks[120]. The 3 monosaccharides are fructose, glucose and galactose.

1. Disaccharides are double sugar molecules. The most common that you may be familiar with already are lactose and sucrose. They cannot be directly absorbed because they cannot cross cell membranes without being broken down into their monosaccharide building blocks[121.]

    Sucrose, table sugar = glucose + fructose
    Lactose, milk sugar = glucose + galactose
    Maltose = glucose + glucose

2. Polysaccharides are the most common in food sources of dietary carbohydrate for all except very young animals. These are sub-categorised into starch and cellulose.

    a. Starch is one major form of plant glucose storage
    b. Cellulose the other form of plant carbohydrate. It is indigestible by human enzymes, yet plays a very important part in supporting our digestive systems by "feeding" our microflora, or gut bacteria. Cellulose is considered a prebiotic.

3. Oligosaccharides are partially broken-down polysaccharides.

Starch is digestible plant carbohydrate. There are three types of starch: rapidly digestible starch, slowly digestible starch and resistant starch.

---

120 http://www.vivo.colostate.edu/hbooks/pathphys/digestion/basics/polysac.html

121 This is true when there is no increased gut permeability in play which can result in disaccharides crossing the membrane into blood where they can cause further problems.

Resistant starch is considered a form of dietary fibre because it is unaffected by digestive enzymes and ferments in the large intestine. This fermentation may cause discomfort from the gases produced. Rapid and slowly digestible starches need high levels of amylase to breakdown the complex sugars.

If you think about the amount of saliva mixing with food in the mouth, is it enough to fully breakdown the volume and complexity of sugars consumed? The answer is no. Rarely do infants mix food sufficiently with saliva to breakdown the starches they eat. And so, given that infants only produce amylase in the mouth and it stops working in stomach acid, complex sugars are not sufficiently broken down to be absorbed. These ferment in the intestine forming gas, and causing trapped wind, bloating, abdominal distention, pain and abdominal tenderness.

Cellulose is a fibre and gives plants their structural integrity. It too is unaffected by human digestive enzymes but does not ferment like resistant starch, so is rarely a source of abdominal discomfort. As a prebiotic, it supports the growth and development of healthy gut bacteria.

You can think of cellulose as insoluble fibre, and resistant starch as water soluble. Starches will remove water from the body as they pass through the digestive system, as well as fermenting. A side effect of these can be constipation and hard stools. On the other hand, plant-based insoluble fibre does not absorb more water from the gut. While feeding the good gut bacteria, it also stimulates peristalsis action in the gut and supports the formation of soft and passable stools.

For infants, I recommend avoiding all starches until pancreatic enzymes have start to be produced effectively, and to have a good intake of fibrous vegetables.

DIETARY SOURCES OF CARBOHYDRATES

The sources of carbs that provide your baby with amazing nutrition as well as being less likely to cause reflux flares include:

Vegetables:

- asparagus
- aubergine (eggplant)
- beetroot
- bell peppers (capsicum)
- broccoli
- Brussels sprouts
- cabbages
- cauliflowers
- carrots
- celery
- courgette (zucchini)
- garlic
- leaves – spinach, lettuces
- mushrooms
- onion
- pumpkins
- squashes – butternut, acorn, spaghetti, queen.

Fruit (always fully ripe):

- avocado
- banana
- coconut
- grapes (seedless)
- mango
- papaya
- pineapple.

8.3.4   PROTEIN

Protein is a crucial food group for your baby. Like carbohydrates, there are simple and complex proteins, some easier, some harder for immature digestive systems to break down. Unlike fat, protein can ferment in the gut.

The simplest form of protein is an amino acid. Proteins most often occur as large molecules made up of one or more chains of amino acids. The digestive process requires the separation and deconstruction of the complex chains into individual amino acids so the body can use them.

As baby has limited pancreatic enzyme production in the first 2 years, most protein digestion is done in the stomach. This means that there is one shot at breaking down proteins. Therefore, the simpler the protein, the easier the digestion, and the lower the risk of fermentation and irritation further down the digestive tract.

Casein, the protein in cow's milk, is a complex protein which may explain why CMPA occurs in infants, and why they mostly grow out of it when their body naturally starts to produce the enzymes that can break down proteins.

Complex proteins should be avoided in infancy until baby has developed their natural ability to digest these foods correctly, rather than misidentifying the proteins as problematic irritants and taking protective action (allergies).

Therefore, careful selection of the correct proteins is important for infant feeding. This will avoid unnecessary reactions, limit allergenic responses and allow your baby to extract the nutrition from the proteins they eat.

Protein is not needed in massive amounts. Remember, the calorific value is the same as carbs, roughly 4 kCal per gram of protein.

Simple proteins for babies include:

- chicken
- dairy produce if tolerated, for example, cheese

- egg white (may be too complex for some babies and can vary in tolerance depending on how it is cooked)
- lamb
- nut products
- oily fish
- pork
- turkey.

8.4   THE MICROS

Micronutrients are the building blocks that our bodies need to perform all their functions. There are hundreds of minerals and vitamins that we require. Some of the most important micronutrients for babies are listed below, including why the body needs them, where to find them, and what the impact of deficiency may be.

Most formula milks are especially designed to ensure they include all the nutrients your baby needs.

8.4.1   IRON

Iron is the micronutrient that enables the blood to carry oxygen around the body. Iron is required for haemoglobin (red blood cells) and a deficiency in iron causes anaemia. It is vital for normal brain development in babies.

If your baby doesn't have enough iron, thay might be pale, gaining weight slowly (dropping down the centile curves), be irritable, fussy and cranky, and have poor appetite. Ongoing iron deficiency will result in slower overall development, poor academic performance with a short attention span and problems concentrating.

Iron is a vital mineral required for proper central nervous system development. In fact, an iron deficiency in babies between 6 and 12 months can impact cognitive and motor and social development skills well into teen years[122].

Babies are born with a reserve of iron, and indeed, delayed cutting of the umbilical cord at birth increases the reserve of iron-rich blood. Breastfed babies continue getting iron through breastmilk.

Once the child is getting their iron intake from food sources, parents should be aware that not all sources of iron are equally readily accessible by the body. Proper intake of iron from food is vital for babies after 6 months. While breastfed babies get iron through breastmilk, most formulas are now fortified with iron. However, the two are not totally comparable. In breastmilk, the iron is solely available for the baby, so it will not feed unfriendly gut bacteria. This is not the case with iron-fortified foods. Pay careful attention to the iron source.

Good sources of iron for babies and toddlers include:

- breastmilk
- winter squash and pumpkins
- meat and poultry (beef, beef liver, chicken liver, turkey, chicken, pork, lamb, lamb liver)
- mushrooms
- greens (spinach, chard, dandelion, beet, parsley)
- nutritional yeast
- egg yolks
- tomatoes
- sardines.

8.4.2   CALCIUM

Calcium is an age-old favourite mineral that has driven mass consumption of dairy products, and makes parents of dairy-intolerance babies panic. The diagnosis of "dairy allergy or intolerance" sets off all

---

122 https://www.ncbi.nlm.nih.gov/pmc/articles/PMC1540447/

sorts of unnecessary alarm bells. *Where will my child get calcium from? All her bones are going to grow wrong. She'll get rickets and break her legs all the time!*

I'm here to tell you that dairy products are not the be all and end all when it comes to calcium needs for your child.

Calcium is not only essential for good bone development, but also for blood to clot, nerves to send messages and muscles to contract. Yet calcium on its own is useless. In fact, without sufficient magnesium and vitamin D, the calcium consumed cannot be effectively absorbed. The greater your intake of vitamin D and magnesium, the less calcium you need to consume because your body will be able to absorb more from what you have consumed. Follow?!

Recommended daily allowances (RDAs) of calcium have been heavily influenced by the dairy industry and are not necessarily the true needs of the body. The calcium RDA we tend to see on packaging is the recommend intake of dairy-based calcium to allow our body to absorb the calcium it needs. However, not all the calcium in dairy is able to be absorbed by our bodies. For dairy products, the calcium is about 30-35% bioavailable.

Children have a dairy requirement of about 700mg per day between 1 and 3 years of age. This is easily achievable with non-dairy based foods. Obviously, if your child does not suffer with a dairy intolerance, cheese, unsweetened yogurts, butter and cream make for great nutritional choices.

Calcium is highest in dairy products. However, there are other non-dairy sources of calcium:

- seeds (chia, sesame, poppy and sesame – suitable for toddlers)
- sardines and canned salmon (because of the bones)
- almonds
- leafy greens (spinach, kale, collards, bok choi)
- rhubarb
- oranges.

8.4.3 CHOLINE

Choline is neither a mineral nor a vitamin, but was recognised by the Institute of Medicine in 1998 as an essential micronutrient, although it still does not have a recommended daily allowance. This water-soluble nutrient plays an important part in the development of the brain and memory, and decreases the risk of neural tube defects in the foetus. It is required for proper brain and liver function, muscle movement and nerve function and supports energy levels and the body's metabolism[123].

Because of the incredible amount of brain development in infants and babies, I believe that we should make sure that our children are getting adequate intake of choline in the early years. "Some reports even show that choline can help prevent learning disabilities, including ADHD, and can improve concentration in children and teens."[120]

The best sources of choline are:

- egg yolks
- beef liver
- salmon
- beef
- turkey
- chicken
- cauliflower
- goats milk
- Brussels sprouts.

8.4.4 VITAMIN A

Vitamin A is a critical nutrient for healthy eye development and eyesight, healthy skin and neurological function. Deficiency in vitamin A can result in night-blindness and total blindness, and increase the risk of disease and death from severe infections.

---

123 https://draxe.com/what-is-choline/

Often orange in colour, the best vitamin A food sources are:

- liver
- potatoes
- carrots
- kale
- spinach
- apricots
- broccoli
- butter
- eggs
- butternut squash.

8.4.5   B VITAMINS

The B vitamins are a class of water-soluble vitamins needed for cell metabolism. While we generally hear a lot about B vitamins, we rarely know what they are for. Here is a summary table for the B vitamins.

Vitamin B name	Why it's needed	Some deficiencies cause
Vitamin B1, thiamine	It plays a central role in the release of energy from carbohydrates. It is involved in DNA production, as well as nerve function	Beriberi, disease of the nervous system, weight loss, emotional disturbances, impaired sensory perception, weakness and pain in the limbs, irregular heartbeat, and oedema
Vitamin B2, riboflavin	Is involved in release of energy from food	cracked lips, high sensitivity to sunlight, inflammation of the tongue, seborrheic dermatitis, sore throat
Vitamin B3, niacin (nicotinic acid), nicotinamide riboside	It play an important role in energy transfer reactions in the metabolism of glucose and fat.	Aggression, dermatitis, insomnia, weakness, mental confusion, and diarrhoea.
Vitamin B5, pantothenic acid	Is needed for the oxidation of fatty acids and carbohydrates.	acne and paresthesia, although it is uncommon.
Vitamin B6, pyridoxine,	Is used in amino acid metabolism	pink eye, neurological symptoms (e.g. epilepsy)

pyridoxal, pyridoxamine		
Vitamin B7, biotin	Food breakdown and absorption	"may lead to impaired growth and neurological disorders in infants."
Vitamin B9, folate	Folate is involved in the transfer of single-carbon units in the metabolism of nucleic acids and amino acids. and is needed for normal cell division, especially during pregnancy and infancy, which are times of rapid growth.	Anaemia, and elevated levels of homocysteine. Deficiency in pregnant women can lead to birth defects.
Vitamin B12	It is essential in the production of blood cells in bone marrow, and for nerve sheaths and proteins.	Anaemia, peripheral neuropathy, memory loss and other cognitive deficits.

We know that generally a well-balanced diet of *fresh* food will be enough to make sure your baby has enough of each.

Good sources of B vitamins include:

- Meat, poultry and fish
- Eggs
- Dairy produce
- Fruit
  - tomatoes
- Vegetables
  - asparagus
  - broccoli
  - Brussels sprouts
  - spinach.

8.4.6   Vitamin C

A common vitamin, but for what? The body cannot grow, repair or heal itself without vitamin C. Given the hidden trauma that can occur for reflux babies or babies with food intolerances, I believe vitamin C is vital to help their bodies heal any inflammation caused by intolerance to foods when irritation in the digestive system is passed to other parts of the body – skin, lungs etc. And the body seeks to heal itself so let's make sure that baby's got the tools and materials to do the necessary repairs.

Good sources of vitamin C for your baby include:

- Fruit
    - mango
    - oranges
    - papaya
    - pineapple
    - tomatoes
- Vegetables
    - bell peppers (capsicum)
    - broccoli
    - Brussels sprouts
    - kale.

8.4.7   VITAMIN D

Required for absorption of calcium and phosphorus, it is necessary for strong teeth and bones, regulates the immune system and is a protective agent against cancer, type 1 diabetes and multiple sclerosis.

The best source is the sun, which needs exposed skin during high sunshine. Some food sources containing vitamin D are:

- oily fish (salmon, mackerel, sardines)
- red meat
- liver
- milk, cow, goat or sheep
- egg yolks.

8.4.8   MAGNESIUM

Magnesium is an essential mineral and has multiple important functions including:

- Being required for the absorption of other minerals

- o   calcium
- o   phosphorus
- o   sodium
- o   potassium
- Being required for the use of some vitamins
  - o   B vitamins
  - o   vitamin C
  - o   vitamin E
- Being used in essential metabolic processes
  - o   activation of enzymes needed to breakdown carbohydrates and proteins
  - o   release of energy from glucose
  - o   synthesis of protein and nucleic acids
  - o   proper formation of urea
  - o   vascular tone (blood vessels)
  - o   efficient muscle action
  - o   electrical stability of the cells
  - o   neurotransmission.

It is easy to see why magnesium is such an important mineral. The greatest danger is posed to children on gastric acid medications which inhibit the effective take-up of magnesium. Without magnesium, the body cannot properly absorb vitamin D and calcium, which can result in rickets along with other bone deficiency diseases.

The best sources of magnesium are:

- breastmilk
- fresh green vegetables
- dairy produce
- seafood
- figs
- apples
- oil-rich nuts and seeds especially almonds (as smooth butters and ground nuts)

- garlic
- peaches and apricots.

You can also add Epsom salts into bathwater, as magnesium is effectively absorbed through the skin.

8.5   FOODS TO AVOID

8.5.1   FATS

Avoid any processed or damaged fats including sunflower oil, canola oil, rapeseed oil. Also avoid hydrogenated fats, trans fats, any fat that has been heated to a high temperature – oils used in deep frying, especially as these oils are often used for many days repeatedly, which damages the oils further.

8.5.2   CARBOHYDRATES

Avoid feeding your child all disaccharides, starch and water-soluble fibre. These groups include apples, pears, all unripe fruit, and all seedy fruit including strawberries, tomatoes, kiwi, melons. Starches include potatoes, sweet potatoes, turnip, swede, parsnip.

Water-soluble fibre includes all grain products, whole grains in porridges or ground flours, wheat, rye, oats, rice, amaranth, sweetcorn. And disaccharides include table sugar, brown sugar (any variety), molasses, agave nectar, maple syrup, coconut sugar, maple sugar, any fruit-based sweetener.

There is only one sweetener that your baby can digest easily: honey. This is safe only after 12 months of age.

Furthermore, avoid concentrated sugars occurring in dried fruits. While infants may have the amylase necessary to break down the sugars in these foods, often the food does not get sufficiently mixed with amylase in the mouth to digest the sugars well enough; some undigested sugars remain.

WHEAT

As a water-soluble food, wheat flour removes water from the body and can play a part in constipation. Gluten can stick to and coat the inside of the intestine, reducing nutrient absorption. Gluten protein is also a complex protein that has high allergenic properties and the sugars in wheat are complex; they simply cannot be digested effectively by your baby. If your baby cannot digest the food then they cannot extract the nutrients from it. While they cannot digest it and their digestive system is growing and maturing, avoid all wheat.

RICE

Breastfeeding mums and children under 5 years should not eat rice as it has a high concentration of arsenic. This arsenic is naturally occurring, yet still poses a threat to the development of a young child. The concentrations as compared with child's body weight are deemed too high to be safe. Arsenic affects cognitive development, as well as general growth and the immune system[124].

The research around rice is ongoing and at present there is no recommended "safe" exposure limit for babies and breastfeeding mothers. A recent survey recommended that parents remove rice from babies' diets to limit and reduce exposure[125].

At present, my advice is to research the brands you wish to purchase or stop altogether. If your child is regularly consuming rice products, the arsenic will cycle out of body in a few days after stopping.

Avoid all puffed rice products and rice cakes. Like many "white products", puffed rice has reduced nutritional content, and while easy and convenient, they are non-local to our environment nor typical staple foods in Western diets. For Eastern locations, there may be an argument that children can tolerate higher levels of arsenic naturally occurring in food

124 https://www.theguardian.com/lifeandstyle/2017/may/04/inorganic-arsenic-rice-cakes-babies-queens-university-belfast
125 Jane Houlihan, MSCE, Healthy Babies Bright Futures http://www.healthybabycereals.org/sites/default/files/2017-12/ HBBF_ArsenicInInfantCerealReport.pdf

produced locally (not for mass market) since it may be processed differently to reduce the arsenic content.

Not for children under 2 years. For children over 2 years, prepare small portions of white rice (not brown rice). Rinse well before cooking fully. Do not freeze or reheat rice due to the increased risk of food poisoning.

A great alternative to rice is cauliflower rice, which has a higher nutritional density and can be used as a direct replacement for rice in risottos, fried and boiled rice dishes.

OATS/PORRIDGE

Often presented as a good baby food, the starch is too much in oats for baby to digest. Soaking oats can make them more digestible and remove some of the indigestible starch. Soaked oats can be introduced gradually after 18 months.

8.5.3   PROTEINS

Avoid complex proteins until your baby's digestive system is producing the pancreatic enzymes to support complex protein digestion in the small intestine. Improperly digested proteins can trigger allergic reactions to "safe" foods, and can also ferment in the gut resulting in gas production that causes bloating and discomfort.

If your child has CMPA, beef and veal meats are also a no-go. You may find that your baby can tolerate dairy products, but reacts to beef because it is a particularly complex protein to digest.

The following proteins should be avoided in infancy (before child has milk teeth):

- beef, veal and all dairy products CMPA present
- shellfish including, but not limited to:
    o   crab
    o   crayfish
    o   lobster
    o   mussels

- oysters
- prawns
- scallops
- shrimp
- raw fish (e.g. sushi)
- smoked fish.

8.5.4   COMBINED CARBOHYDRATE AND PROTEINS

Although we know these substances to be nutritious in adults, your young baby does not have the ability to digest the combination of carbohydrate and protein in plant sources properly. Vegetable proteins from legumes should also be avoided in infancy (before child has all milk teeth); they are protected by nature with inhibitors (phytic acid). This applies to all legumes including beans, lentils, lupins, peanuts, peas and pulses.

Some of the legumes you may be familiar with that you will need to avoid for your baby initially include:

- beans
  - haricot (as in baked beans)
  - broad beans
  - butter beans
  - flat beans
  - green beans
  - kidney beans
  - lima beans
  - mung beans
  - navy beans
  - soy beans
  - runner beans
- peas
  - black-eyed peas
  - field peas
  - garden peas
  - snap peas

     o   snow peas

     o   split peas

- chickpeas
- lentils
- lupins.

The above list is not exhaustive. All legumes should be avoided. You may, of course, find out that your baby is okay with some of these, but your baby will be an exception to the rule rather than the rule here.

8.5.5   PHYTIC ACID/WHOLE FOODS

Phytic acid is how several grains, seeds and nuts store phosphorus. Humans do not have the enzymes required to break it down and it can cause problems as a result. In addition, it binds to essential minerals such as calcium, iron and magnesium so that they cannot be absorbed. The presence of phytic acid could lead to a deficiency of these minerals.

Avoid whole nuts and seeds because your baby's digestive system has a hard time breaking down the outside plant cell walls, which are not broken by chewing, meaning digestive enzymes cannot access the food inside the seeds.

While most seeds are large and not offered to baby (e.g. sunflower and pumpkin seeds), some are so small that they do not pose a choking hazard and are often found in food for children. These seeds include poppy, sesame, strawberry, tomato, kiwi, melon, pomegranate, passionfruit, figs, starfruit, dragonfruit. Take good care with raspberries, blueberries, cranberries, blackberries and currants which have small seeds within them. I have found that children over 12 months better tolerate riper fruits in small quantities.

8.6   FOODS TO NEVER GIVE BABY

There are some foods that I believe we should all stay away from. Here are my top three no-no foods:

- Margarine/vegetable oil spreads – vegetable oils that are liquid by nature become solid at room temperature with hydrogenised fat. And just because your granny used it doesn't make it healthy. The human body recognises trans fats as dangerous and as such uses naturally produced cholesterol to lock it away before it harms our body. Too much trans fat in the body causes circulating cholesterol levels to increase, which causes problems as it exceeds a saturation point, sticking to arteries and clogging the system. Not how to have a happy body. Use cold-pressed or expeller-pressed oils that are naturally solid at room temperature like coconut oil instead.

- Canola/rapeseed oil – touted as the new "heat-resistant" healthy cooking oil, this is far from the truth. This oil, particularly in the US, has been so heavily genetically modified and over-processed with heat that it doesn't bear any resemblance to a healthy cooking oil. Just because it looks a lovely golden yellow colour doesn't mean it's healthy.

- Sugar – this plays havoc with baby's microbiome and there is no reason on earth that baby needs white sugar. There are plenty of naturally occurring sugars that give baby sweetness as well as nutrition – fruit, honey, maple syrup.

8.7   FOODS TO EAT

The list of foods infants can eat is long and varied. It provides a fabulous base for many nutritious and tasty meals. Below is my list of safe foods. However, you must remember that every food is a ***potential irritant or allergen*** and observe reactions to everything you feed your child.

In my view, ideal foods for baby are high in saturated fats, the fats required for brain development, such as egg yolks and ripe avocado. Also start by trying ripe bananas and squashes. ***This is enough food for baby to be eating for the first few weeks***.

Remember, for the first few months, food is about familiarising your little one with eating. Babies at this stage are learning how to use their mouth, tongue and digestive system to digest solid food. Baby needs to learn these skills consciously or unconsciously, as they give baby the foundation of a healthy life.

The next table lists foods most easily digested by an infant's gradually maturing digestive system, nutritious and wholesome.

Fats	Animal produce
	egg yolks
	dairy —butter, cream, yogurt
	goat and sheep cheeses, creams & yogurts
	Meat, opting for grass-fed and preferably organic
	ground meat (has a great high fat content, beef
	pork
	veal
	lamb
	Poultry
	goose fat
	duck fat
	Oily fish
	salmon
	mackerel
	trout
	sardines
	herring
	tuna
	Fruit
	avocados
	coconuts – oil, milk, cream and flesh
	coconut yogurt
	olives
	Nuts (as ground or milled nuts, flours or smooth butters)
	almonds
	brazil nuts

	cashews
	macadamia
	pecans
	walnuts
	Seeds
	cocoa butter
	chia seeds, meal or ground
	ground flaxseed
	Oils (vegetable oils should be cold pressed)
	olive oil
	flax oil (never heat)
	coconut oil
	goose fat, duck fat
Carbohydrates	Fruit (all fruit should be **fully** ripe)
	banana
	blackberries
	blueberries (cut open)
	grapes (cut lengthways)
	mango
	papaya
	pineapple
	raspberries
	tomato flesh
	Vegetables
	bell peppers (capsicum)
	broccoli – calabrese, sprouting and purple
	broccoflowers (broccoli cauliflower hybrids)
	carrots
	cauliflowers (including snowball (regular) and romanesco)
	garlic
	herbs – coriander, parsley, mint, thyme, rosemary, sage
	leafy greens – cabbage, spinach, lettuces, beet leaves, chard, Brussels sprouts
	mushrooms
	onion
	pumpkins
	squashes (summer – courgette/zucchini, winter – butternut, coquina, acorn etc)
	Animal produce
	milk (cow or goat)
Proteins	Chicken (organic, free range)

Turkey

Pork

Lamb

Beef

Salmon

Cod

Haddock

Tuna* (caution with mercury content)

Egg white (if well tolerated)

* Take care with the volume of tuna you give young children due to the high levels of mercury.

8.7.1   CHOOSING FRUIT

Ripeness in fruit is an extremely important aspect to support digestion. An unripe banana is crunchier and has more starch compared to a ripe banana. Starch, you will remember, will irritate your baby's digestive system, causing pain and bloating. A ripe banana, is soft and squishy, essentially the ripening process has converted the starches to sugars all by itself! Amazing! The ripe one is what your baby needs. Always make sure the stalk has no green left on it and the skin of the banana is starting to speckle with black dots.

A ripe avocado is another of nature's natural convenience foods. They are jam-packed full of goodness. Make sure that avocado being offered to your baby is ripe, even over-ripe. It should be soft and give with a little pressure. When you remove the stalk the inside should be green to black (yellow under the stalk means the avocado is not ripe so do not open it yet). The stone should be easily removable and come away from the flesh cleanly. A spoon or blunt knife should pass through the flesh easily. There should be no need for a sharp knife to cut the avocado flesh.

Tropical fruits are usually a bright colour on the skin when ripe. Mangoes should be red-orange with no green skin; pineapples should be golden yellow in colour; papaya should be a rosy orange.

Pineapple, mango and papaya are great fruits to boost digestion in infants, because in their ripe and raw form they contain natural digestive enzymes. The foods themselves are easily digested by baby's immature digestive system.

8.8   Common Allergenic Foods

The truth is that every single food and substance on this planet has the capacity to be an allergen. An awareness of how allergic reactions present is therefore what's required. You must be able to spot allergic reactions and know what your baby is exposed to so that you can identify the source.

The table of foods and substances is a reference point of common allergens that have a documented history of allergenic response (IgE response). This list does not reflect a maturing digestive system. Remember, allergens are not the same as irritants to an immature digestive system; however, babies can grow out of both.

This table is a guideline for reference only.

Least allergenic substances	Animal products
	chicken
	pork
	lamb
	salmon
	turkey
	Grains
	rice
	millet
	quinoa (although technically a seed)
	Fruit
	apples
	avocado
	apricots
	banana
	blueberries
	dates
	grapes
	mango
	papaya

	peaches
	pears
	raisins
	raspberries
	Vegetables
	beetroot
	broccoli
	carrot
	cauliflower
	broccoli
	lettuce
	squash
	courgette
	sweet potato
	potato
	swede
	turnip
	parsnip
	celeriac
	bell peppers
	cucumber
	cabbage
	onions
	garlic
	leeks
Most highly allergenic substances	Animal products
	dairy including beef
	egg whites
	fish – e.g. cod
	shellfish
	Grains
	gluten (including wheat, oats, barley)
	soy products (including soya)
	corn (including maize and polenta)
	buckwheat
	Nuts and seeds
	peanuts
	tree nuts (walnut, almond, pecan)
	sesame
	Fruit

	strawberries
	kiwi
	citrus fruits
	tomatoes
	Additives and preservatives
	sulphur – appears as sulphur dioxide, sulphates and sulphites (used in foods as preservatives and in bathing products)
	food dyes such as tartrazine, annatto, and carmine
Other non-food allergens	Pet dander
	Dust and dust mites
	Mould spores
	Mosquito bites
	Bee stings
	Parabens (also found in bathing products – identify on labels as ethyl-, methyl-, propyl- or butyl-paraben)

Refer to section 3.1 Symptoms: What To Look For (page 30). for a list of symptoms that may indicate an allergic or irritation response.

9   FOUNDATIONS OF CHANGE

If you have figured out that your baby is likely to be reacting to something in their milk or food, you must track down the likely culprit(s), eliminate them, get your baby to their Place of Great and keep them there while you rebuild their diet.

I have a few tools to help you do this, regardless of how your baby is currently fed. For additional breastfeeding resource, see chapter 10 The Breastfeeding Protocol (page199).

9.1   PLACE OF GREAT

This is where we want your baby to get to – their Place of Great. This will be different for every baby, so it is important that you define what this looks like for your baby.

Some examples of what a Place of Great might be for particular babies are:

a) A baby who struggles with constant abdominal pain, wind, constipation, poor sleep, irritable and cranky all the time with a bowel movement only once a week; their Place of Great could simply be "no longer constipated", because many of the other symptoms are associated with this one.

b) A baby who spends every afternoon thrashing about in agony, screaming and crying, arching their back, impossible to hold and impossible to comfort. Their Place of Great is more about not being in pain any longer, and every afternoon is settled, happy and contented, just as they are in the morning.

c) A baby who is mostly fine during the day, sleeps in a carrier and loves to be held and comforted, but turns into a different child once 7pm has passed. This might look like baby only settling in arms, cannot be put down. Bedtime takes up to 3 hours, sometimes more. Baby wakes 8-12 times every night, suckles to go back to sleep, or wakes at 1am screaming, and does not settle for up to 3 hours until that wind has passed, and is in agony waiting for it. Then once 7am comes, they are a beautiful baby once again. Their Place of Great is more about not having painful trapped wind to deal with, and waking during the night is not a problem if it only takes them 5 minutes to settle again.

These three scenarios by no means describe half of the unsettled babies out there; they serve to highlight how different a Place of Great for any baby will be, because reflux pain is experienced so differently; it will also be influenced by how mum and dad feel in all this.

9.2   Journaling for Success

Here are some tips to provide you with the support you may need on your journey. The goal is to get your baby to a place of happier and more settled as quickly as possible, and then start reintroducing foods into your / their diet in a safe and controlled way, identifying and avoiding any irritants.

1. Journal how you feel right now before you start. Write a detailed letter to yourself about the pain you are experiencing, the lack of sleep, how hard the nights are, the dread you feel when bedtime approaches. For me, this looked like facing 12 hours of loneliness every night. Re-read this letter whenever you are tempted by convenience, (e.g. buying the pre-made baby foods, or tempted by the food you have eliminated), remind yourself how bad it was and take stock of improvements made so far.

2. Willpower and determination are key for an elimination diet (even if you are not doing it but just managing your baby's food).

   To make sure you have these in spades, write down *why* you want to do this, why it is important and what results you want to achieve from the change. Any time you are feeling deflated, re-read these reasons. When these reasons are bigger than you, you are more likely to stick to your diet. (For example, when it is for your baby's health and wellbeing, this is a "bigger than you" reason to do something.)

3. If your wee one doesn't sleep at night and you're knackered, adopt a *very* early bedtime. Don't fight the exhaustion. Studies show that our willpower, determination and ability to make good decisions is poor or lacking in the evenings. Therefore, avoid having to make decisions at this time of day. For a few weeks, help yourself out by catching up on sleep. Make your life easier!

4. Set baby's bedtime to 7pm, regardless of any other factors. If you know your baby will be up every hour throughout the night, and until now you've had a bedtime for both of you at 11pm, you are making things worse for you both. All you're doing is changing rooms together. Baby should sleep in the bedroom from 7pm. This can be on your shoulder, in a cot or in your bed, depending on your preferred sleeping pattern. If you have to stay in the room with your little one, that's fine! Shift your bedtime too.

    You may be thinking: *But I won't get to see my husband/partner!* I challenge this. What is the quality of time you have with your partner right now? Are your evenings yours to share or are they more concerned with baby? Would you be better placed to spend time with your partner as a happier mum, after two really early nights and sleep? Would you be on a more even keel and up early in the morning? Would your husband prefer a more emotionally stable wife? Have you the means to watch your favourite TV show in your bed? Would your husband join you for a few early nights? I suggest that the answer to most of these questions is *yes!* Adopt this strategy for 2 weeks and see if there is a positive shift in your life.

5. Diary or journal every morning. Set out your intention. This is a proven method to support you in what you want to achieve. EXAMPLE: *I am going to eat the right food for me and my baby today. I know what I have to do. I can do this. I have the support I need and I do not have to justify this to anyone. I believe in myself. I want to have great sleep. I want my baby to be comfortable. I am confident in what I am trying because it has given me results already.*

    If you can't find the time to write this every morning, write it on a sheet of A4 paper once, and hang this piece of paper by the bathroom mirror so that when you go to brush your teeth/wash your face every morning, you can read it to yourself. Read it aloud. Reinforce your own beliefs. Another idea is to write it on the chalkboard when you're playing with your baby. Have fun with it!

6. Make a food plan and do your shopping. Planning ahead makes it easier to stick to your food regime. Know what you're going to eat and have the food in the house. Make 3-4 portions of a meal so that you have some to stick in the fridge for the next day or freezer for next week.

7. If you are doing an elimination diet, ask your husband/partner to support you by eating the same food when he is at home. This means nobody has to cook two meals and you are not facing temptation at every corner. Ask him to read this part of the book (and the rest of it) so that he too understands what is going on, what you are trying to achieve and how you want to get there. Ask him to positively reinforce everything that you are doing. Ask him to support your evening routine by tidying the kitchen and lounge before he comes to bed so that your morning is chore-free. Do this for 2 weeks and I'm pretty sure your relationship see great improvements too. Your sleep will greatly improve. Your emotional state will greatly improve. Your lives will be calmer, fuller, happier and more connected.

8. Create a visual reward chart for yourself and hang it on the fridge. This may sound trivial and nonsensical, but we use visual reward charts with children to improve behaviour and build new routines all the time. Sometimes it is not enough to know baby is a little better than last week. Visual charts for your own food consumption are powerful in reinforcing your own behaviour over a few weeks. Have a "prize" for 100% compliance, such as your partner committing to be home early on a Friday afternoon to look after baby so you can go for a massage or haircut.

9. After 2 weeks, you will likely see some change if you have stuck to the diet. At this point, you can start adding food back into your diet. If you are still breastfeeding, add food back into your diet first.

    Then if and when baby is on solids, add in foods one at a time for baby too with at least 2 days between, as there may be foods that your digestive system can process but baby cannot. Also remember that baby is not "missing out" on taste or flavour at any stage. Baby is still learning about these. Thinking in the longer term will make it more enjoyable for your wee one, rather than potentially subjecting them to periods of discomfort.

10. If you notice a reaction after a food has been reintroduced, remove the food and do not add anything else back into the diet until all symptoms have completely disappeared again. Once baby is good again, introduce another food.

    Once a breastfed baby is on solids, do not introduce them to a food that has caused a reaction in them when you reintroduced it back into *your* diet.

9.3   SAFE FOODS

Some foods are more easily digestible than others. Understanding how foods are broken down is the foundation of my approach. The foods detailed in this section are specifically for babies who are on solids and getting a substantial portion of their energetic and nutritional requirements from food. If your baby has not yet started solids or is eating only very little, please refer to chapter 11 Introducing Solid Food (page 219).

Always provide baby (or breastfeeding mum) with the whole foods only. Stay away from pouches, juices and dried fruits as the sugars are often more concentrated, causing an overload in baby's system without the fibre that is required to slow absorption and digestion.

9.3.1   VEGETABLES

Yes Veg	No Veg
Broccoli, cauliflower, courgette (zucchini), marrow, winter squash: butternut, spaghetti, acorn, pumpkin, celery, sprouted foods (e.g. bean sprouts), asparagus, beetroot, mushroom, aubergine (eggplant), celery, onion, garlic, butternut squash, bell peppers, carrots, radish	Starches: potato, sweet potato, celeriac, turnip, parsnip, swede, kohlrabi
Green leaves: spinach, salad leaves	Legumes: peas, sweetcorn, beans of any variety, lentils, spilt peas, chickpeas
Vegetable oils: olive oil (expeller cold-pressed only), coconut oil (aroma-free for cooking), flax oil (never heated, only as a salad dressing), avocado oil	Soy, soya and related products (e.g. emulsifiers)

9.3.2   FRUIT

Fruit can be a little more irritant and so limiting fruit for the first 2-3 weeks will serve you well.

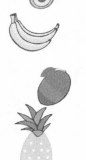

Yes Fruit	No Fruit
Fruit must be ripe to be safe Avocado Banana Olives Plums Peaches Tropical fruit: mango, pineapple, papaya	Any seedy fruit: strawberry, raspberry, blackberry, blueberry, cranberry, black currant, kiwi, melon, grapes Any hard fruit: apple, pear, persimmon Any dried fruit Citrus fruit: lemons, grapefruit, orange, limes

9.3.3   ANIMAL PRODUCE

Animal source foods are amazing sources of protein and healthy fats.

Yes Produce	No Produce
Eggs: egg yolk is safer than white, though it is worth trialling egg white as it provides an amazing base for baking and easy nutritious meals	Dairy of all types: milk, cream, cheese, yogurt, butter, beef, veal, cured meats with additives
Fish: salmon (organic or wild, not smoked), mackerel, herring, sardines, white fish	Egg white to start
Meat: lamb, pork, cured meats with salt and water only	Shellfish: crab, prawns, lobster, crayfish, mussels
Poultry: chicken, turkey, duck, goose	
Gelatin (avoid beef gelatin if there is any suspicion of CMPA)	
Fats: butter and cream (where no milk allergy or intolerance), lard, duck fat, goose fat, suet, tallow, crackling (cooked only in oil with salt)	

For vegetarian and vegan mums, you should make sure you are getting adequate protein and iron intake. You can try some of the following with the awareness that some ingredients within them may upset your baby.

- Quorn – in its simplest form and with an awareness that the egg white may cause disruption.

- Quinoa – pre-soaking for at least 2 hours and rinsing well before cooking will nullify the phytic acid and support digestion.

- Chia seeds – because they are a seed, they may cause upset, but if you find you can already tolerate them well, they may be okay to eat while breastfeeding.

9.3.4   Other Foods

Yes Produce	No Produce
Tree nuts (almonds, walnuts, coconut, macadamia): pre-soak and dehydrate before eating to support digestion. Ground nuts are easier to digest and should be tried before whole nuts	Alcohol (the sugars are too strong), you may find this in baking products such as vanilla extract
Sweeteners: honey	Grains including wheat, oats (porridge)
Spirulina	Peanuts
Herbs: take care as herbs are often either lactogenic or anti-lactogenic so use wisely according to you individual situation	Seeds
	Spices
	Soy/soya products
	Sweeteners: sugar, maple syrup, agave, fruit sweeteners
	Vinegars

9.3.5   Drinks

The best drink for everyone is water! Some herbal teas can be supportive of your and baby's digestive system. You can also get special nursing mum tea blends.

Yes Produce	No Produce
Water	Milk
Herbal teas: ginger, chamomile, peppermint, nursing mum	Alcohol
	Fruit juice
Coconut water	Coffee
Coconut milk	Hot chocolate (commercial varieties)

9.4   INTRODUCING NEW FOODS

When you introduce a new food, follow the guidelines in section 9.4.1 Introducing New Foods (page 195) to minimise flare-ups and give yourself the best chance of identifying potential irritants.

Always get your baby to their Place of Great before introducing new foods. This way you will be able to determine whether a food is causing symptoms.

Keep a list of **safe foods**, foods that you know, without a shred of doubt in your mind, that you have tried with your baby and seen no reaction. This is so important for when you need to take a step back, or when baby has a cold or other symptom that is hanging around. This is your go-to list that will allow you to have complete confidence in the foods you are giving your baby. And it is also your list of foods that you can share with other family members, childcare providers and babysitters to ensure that they do not make mistakes.

At 3 years old, Daffodil still has multiple food allergies. One of them is sulphites, which is a problem because they naturally occur in foods, and manufacturers only have to label foods if there are more than 10 parts per million of sulphites in the food. This is a relatively low concentration of sulphites, unless you have an allergy, when this amount is more than enough to cause a reaction.

My dad took my daughter to a local café for lunch. A place I have vetted and am totally comfortable with her visiting. I said she could have a bottle of apple juice to drink with her lunch, so my dad got her the apple juice. She loved lunch with Granddad.

That night, her breathing was way off, cold-like symptoms were strong even though there was no sign of a runny nose, and she was full of congestion, breathing loudly and starting to wake because she wasn't getting enough air when sleeping. It turns out that the apple juice she had been given was from concentrate.

In allowing her the apple juice, I hadn't been clear enough and she'd drunk a glass of concentrated apple juice, which I know to be highly likely to contain sulphites regardless of labelling. I can only take responsibility for this myself, because I was not explicitly clear about the particular brand (the "safe food") and that no other apple juice was allowed.

The event resulted in me sleeping in her single bed with her to make sure she was breathing all night. I say "sleeping", but it was more like lying with my eyes closed and listening. My worried husband slept poorly. My daughter wasn't breathing properly so had massively disrupted sleep and was way overtired the next morning for preschool. And my poor dad felt awful.

This is the result of not being specific about known safe foods and known allergies. So often, people outside the immediate family do not realise the impact it has on normal functioning of the household. Understanding allergies and intolerances is so important, especially for your own peace of mind. If, and when, others are looking after your child, you must make sure that they support your baby properly.

I have known grandparents to be so blasé and "non-believing" about allergies that they quite happily fed bread to an officially diagnosed coeliac, resulting in horrendous tummy pain and diarrhoea for days. Because they were no longer in the house when the reaction happened, they didn't see it and it wasn't real to them, so the poor parents are left to deal with the consequences. More on this in section 13 Relationships and Reflux (page 257).

9.4.1   Introducing New Foods
To introduce a new food, follow these guidelines:

1. Start from baby's Place of Great.

    Ideally, your baby's Place of Great is symptom-free, although this may not be possible in the beginning. This means your child has a basic diet where you're 100% confident of the foods not causing painful or uncomfortable symptoms.

2. Decide which food you want to introduce. And when you would
    be most prepared to deal with potential negative symptoms.

    If you choose a food from the "likely allergen" group, then
    perform a patch test the night before. If you don't want to be up all
    night, you may try introducing the food at breakfast that morning
    so reactions have a greater chance of showing up during the day. It
    is not guaranteed that morning ingestion of food will be clear from
    the digestive tract by night-time, but there is a greater chance of
    this happening, so that night-time is more settled.

    Alternatively, if you prefer to observe symptoms during the night,
    you may feel the evening meal is a better time to introduce a new
    food.

3. Always introduce the fully cooked food before trying it raw, as
    cooking aids digestion and breakdown of the food.

4. Introduce foods in small quantities first, gradually increasing the
    amount over the next 3 or 4 days if no reaction is observed.

5. Wait 4 days after first introduction to be sure of a clear response.

6. If you observe a negative reaction to the food (no matter how
    mild), stop feeding it immediately.

7. If you observe a reaction that causes immediate and worrying
    respiratory problems, call the emergency services.

8. Do not introduce foods already confirmed as allergens to your
    child without full paediatric supervision. This sort of oral challenge
    (e.g. severe CMPA) is usually done in a hospital under strict
    supervision.

9.4.2   IDENTIFYING AN IRRITANT

To understand what is causing an irritation, you need three things:

1.   Your own observational skills.
2.   Your personal record of what you baby was like in the days before introducing a new food. (This should be their Place of Great.)
3.   The list of potential symptoms in section 3.1 Symptoms: What To Look For (page 30).

Any changes in appearance, settledness or behaviour in your baby can be a result of a food, if the symptom is not easily explainable by other simple circumstances. For example, you may notice that your baby is particularly irritable one afternoon after the reintroduction of a new food in the morning. Some questions you need to ask to determine if this is likely to be attributable to the food are:

1.   Does baby have any other symptoms? For example, new spots on the skin, sneezing more. A combination of symptoms is more likely to be a food-related issue.
2.   Is your baby tired? How was baby's sleep last night? Are naps on target? If baby is tired, you might conclude that the food is not the problem, but you should note it, as it is not definite.
3.   If cold symptoms appear suddenly, ask yourself if your baby has been in contact with anyone with a strong cold recently?
       a.   If yes, this could be a cold, which should start to improve within a few days.
       b.   If your baby is breastfed, the likelihood of catching a cold is much lower due to the immunity your milk provides. If the cold is prolonged (more than a few days), this is a likely food trigger.

If you suspect a food, or if you are not clear that a food is causing irritation, *stop* the food immediately until all symptoms have cleared/improved and your baby is back to their personal Place of Great (even if this is not perfect, back to their baseline). Do not introduce a new food until they have had 2 consecutive days of great. Park the suspect food on a list of "suspected/unclear" until you can try it again and move it to "definite problem" or "safe".

10 THE BREASTFEEDING PROTOCOL

For more detailed information and guidance, please check out the Breastfeeding Course at www.thebabyrefluxlady.co.uk/book-reader

Breastfeeding is the absolute best way of supporting your baby. There are a rare few occasions when this is not possible, and these cases are extremely serious such as Galactosemia and alactasia. However, for most babies, breastfeeding gives them the absolute best start in life.

Society does not do enough to support breastfeeding, by a long way. In the UK it is estimated that only 4% of babies are breastfed for more than 6 weeks. And for those who do wish to continue breastfeeding, it can feel like a battle and a fight. Your belief that you are absolutely doing the best by your baby is often disregarded and belittled by those close to you. Breastfeeding is so often seen as something that is unnecessary. This unhealthy image of breastfeeding is damaging our children's health. It is undermining the health of the nation in 40-60 year's time and it is shown already to be costing the economy billions of pounds in lost revenue due to the

So congratulations on choosing to breastfeed your baby.

Congratulations on choosing to stand firm in your beliefs.

I am horrified when I hear that doctors and midwives are recommending mums switch to formula to support an unsettled baby, be it colic, reflux, silent reflux, food intolerances or allergies.

The reason it upsets me so much is that rarely does formula resolve the reflux. There are ingredients in formula milk that cause more harm than good and the formulas are completely rigid in the ingredients.

The truth is, breastmilk is the most versatile and controllable of all the milk options for your baby along with all the other well-known benefits of it.

You have complete control of the ingredients in breastmilk. Your diet 100% influences the contents of your breastmilk. What also affects the contents of breastmilk is the health of your own digestive system.

Over the coming weeks I hope to share with you the interactions between your body and your baby's'. And what you need to be aware of as a breastfeeding mum to support your baby as best as possible.

Your baby cannot be allergic to your breastmilk. They can, however, react to something in your breastmilk. And it is not always the "allergens" that cause a problem.

I go for BIG results, FAST.

Your baby my primary client.

I want you to feel confident in your ability to make the correct decision for you and your baby at any stage over the next few years.

Whether your baby is eating solids yet or not, if you are breastfeeding and there are signs of abdominal irritation of any sort in your child, or any allergic symptoms, then it is well worth doing an elimination diet yourself.

If your baby is on solids, you will need to do a combined elimination diet of foods you are both eating that may be upsetting your baby's digestive system.

I have created a simple template that tracks food and symptoms. I cannot stress enough how important it is for you to record this information. If you are in any ways tired, you will forget... You will forget just how hard it is sometimes. You will forget just how painful it is to hear your baby's screams. You will forget how things have changed and may think you are not making progress. When you *write it down*, you have a clear indisputable record of what life is like in your shoes right now and a concrete documentation of what your baby is going through.

Detailed information in food and symptom diaries allows you to identify patterns. The challenge with food intolerance is symptoms may not show for several hours and multiple foods may affect your baby, all with different lag times on symptoms.

You can download a free template from my website at https://www.thebabyrefluxlady.co.uk/book-reader

10.1   Why "Elimination Diets" Fail

Some people swear by the Dr Sears Total Elimination Diet and others are confused because even that didn't work for them.

And I'm here to tell you that there is a very simple reason that the TED diet, GAPS, Paleo, vegan, vegetarian, FODMAP, FPIES, MSPI diets and every other 'diet' or way of eating under the sun could 'fail' to give you predictable and consistent results for your breastfed baby. There is one reason and one reason alone.

These diets fail to consider the current stage of maturity of your baby's digestive system.

It is that simple.

That is the answer.

And that is why this way works, regardless of any other food preferences in your life.

I will teach you what you need to know about your baby's digestive system, because armed with this knowledge you can then make informed and better decisions for you and your baby.

To make the greatest impact first, we are going to start with what will bring you and your baby greatest benefit quickest. And that is to resolve their discomfort, as much of it as is humanly possible. In most cases, I hope that is all of it.

10.2   A DIFFERENT APPROACH

My approach differs from many other breastfeeding elimination diets.

First, you need to understand what is causing your baby's discomfort.

When it comes to food, I take account of the natural immaturity of your baby's digestive system and combine that with a knowledge of the molecular level of the food when digested. This is not taken into account by mainstream practice at present for addressing reflux and infant allergies. This interaction can be the singular source of discomfort, and explains why your baby will "grow out" of these intolerances. It is actually that their digestive system matures to be able to break them down.

I do not propose a single list of safe foods and stick with them for as long as your breastfeeding journey continues.

I start with a massive elimination diet, having the safest of safe foods included. Note that there is no guarantee that any food is 100% "safe", as *anyone* of us has the potential to react to *anything*. The aim here is to remove all allergens, complex proteins and complex carbohydrates immediately. You should start to see improvement in your baby in days.

The approach then is to reintroduce foods in a measured and safe way.

I want you to be able to understand all the range of foods that you can enjoy and understand what you should stay away from for the moment and why. I want you to have the confidence in your choices. I want you to be able to go out to your local pub for lunch and order food you know is not going to bring back the Night from Hell for your little bundle.

So this really becomes an evolving way of eating to support your breastfed baby, and as they grow and develop, you have to confidence and knowledge to introduce more foods gradually and safely. You deserve to be able to enjoy parenthood with ease and that's my goal for you.

10.3   HOW-TO'S FOR SUCCESS

For the breastfeeding elimination diet, you can choose to eliminate foods gradually or completely. I outline the differences between them in this table, but recommend the complete elimination diet for faster results. You will rebuild your diet faster too. This is often reason enough to support the willpower and determination required for these diets!

	Complete Elimination Diet	Gradual elimination of foods
Pros	Quickest route to a complete solution for you and baby Clear outcomes Quick results to improve life, sleep, emotions	Easier on the mental side to gradually drop food from diet Feel like you can continue with life eating "normally" Slower depletion of willpower during the day
Cons	Other people won't understand and will try to tempt you to "give in" Temptation to introduce foods too fast High risk of assuming only one food is the culprit and after discovering one food, then overloading your system and baby's	May not see results for weeks depending on what you drop from your diet High risk of giving up totally and being disheartened by the lack of results Other people not understanding what you are trying to achieve and using the lack of results or slow progress to reinforce the lack of belief in what you're doing
Requires	Determination willpower support planning	Less willpower much longer time less planning

For breastfeeding mums, the complete elimination diet requires a little more willpower, but the results are far quicker both in identifying problem foods and rebuilding your diet to a greatly varied and enjoyable one.

As a breastfeeding mum, follow this diet for 2 weeks and note the changes. Then follow the rules to introduce new foods as outlined in section 9.4.1 Introducing New Foods 195). The same rules apply. Wait 4 days between new foods, if you see symptoms in your baby, stop that food.

If your baby is already eating solids, you must do the elimination diet for you both simultaneously. There are a few rules that will support you both getting to that Place of Great quickly:

1. At the start, eat the same food as your baby each day. You can have the "whole" food if your baby is eating purees. For example, baby might have avocado puree for breakfast, you can have slices of avocado and can add in something like chicken that baby will be having for lunch.
2. If you notice a reaction in your own body, stop eating the food. Your baby may not react to it, but there is a higher chance of reaction. It is also beneficial for you to not be managing symptoms in your own body.
3. If you notice a reaction in your baby, stop that food for you both.
4. When introducing foods, introduce to your baby first. If they have no reaction, you can safely eat that food and breastfeed.

10.3.1   THE ORIGINS OF ELIMINATION

The original Total Elimination Diet (TED) was developed by Dr Crook in 1984. Where this TED fails is that it completely ignores the digestive developmental stages of your baby. There are foods used on the TED that your baby simply cannot digest, and so if you have tried it as a breastfeeding mum and it did not work, there is a reason why that may be the case.

This also applies to virtually all of the "alternate" ways of eating – Gut and Psychology Syndrome Diet (GAPS), Low-FODMAP (Fermentable Oligosaccharides, Disaccharides, Monosaccharides and Polyols), Food Protein-Induced Enterocolitis Syndrome (FPIES) safe foods. The food types in these diets are not completely supportive of the infant digestive system. In fact, when it comes to a FPIES diagnosis, this does not surprise me, and I think all of the foods safe in my way of feeding babies are aligned to FPIES. This is, in my belief however, something that babies naturally grow out of given their continuing digestive development.

10.3.2   STRATEGY FOR SUCCESS

If your baby is not breastfed, then you only need to record what foods they are consuming. You should also look at the ingredients in the formula milk they are drinking and revisit latch on the bottle depending on the symptoms they are showing.

To succeed with an elimination diet, there are a few rules you should always follow:

1. Before you start, write down how your baby is, their level of pain, your feelings about it, how long it takes them to settle. Everything.
2. Record absolutely every last detail.
3. Only make one change at a time, otherwise you will not be able to track down where the results are coming from. During the first 2-week period of an elimination diet, do not do anything else. Postpone complementary or alternative care appointments, maintain medication doses.
4. If you have a mishap and it all goes pear-shaped, start again. This might happen if you go away for the weekend, for example. Pick up where you left off, not the complete beginning. And always get your baby back to a "Place of Great" before introducing more foods.
5. Plan ahead. Draw up a meal plan and know what (you and) your baby are going to eat over the next few weeks. Do your shopping accordingly.
6. If your baby is on medication, you should have an awareness of any possible side effects that are symptoms you wish to eliminate.
7. The younger your baby, the less fussy they will be about wanting variety of food.
8. Talk to your baby about the process, why you are reducing the variety of foods they eat and what you hope to achieve for them.

Do not underestimate the power of communication or what your baby can understand.

9. If you notice a reaction in your baby, stop that food immediately regardless of how minor the reaction.

10. Take it slowly and gently.

11. Remove your need for variety in food from your baby. Step out of your head when it comes to introducing solid food to them.

10.4   ASSUMPTIONS

This diet considers all the nuances of your baby's digestive development, and assumes that your body is functioning properly.

In particular, be aware if you suffer from any digestion-related irritation, because you'll need to be extra careful with your diet for your baby. If you have digestive complaints, you are likely to have increased intestinal permeability, which means that complex sugars and partially undigested foods are passing into your bloodstream and into your milk. If these particles contain complex sugars, this may irritate your baby because your baby cannot digest these foods. (See Section 8 Food for Babies page 145 for details).

The aim is to get your baby to a happier more settled place as quickly as possible.

For 3 weeks, eat only foods that are on the lists above as 'Yes' foods. For best results, limit your diet to as few foods as reasonably possible to start with, this will give you the greatest chance of success for your baby's digestive system to recover.

10.5   TWO METHODS

For the breastfeeding mum's elimination diet, you can do two variants – complete elimination that starts with very low variety of food and gradually builds up to a greatly varied diet or partial elimination that has a much greater variety of food in the beginning and carries some low-level risk of maintaining some intolerances for baby.

Whichever you choose, keep your food and symptom diary, and use that as your ongoing reference point.

With all foods, if you have an allergy or intolerance to a particular food yourself, **do not** consume it regardless of whether or not it is in the elimination diet. These diets **must** be tailored to your individual needs and the examples set out in this section do not consider personal circumstances.

Personally, I do not recommend a gradual elimination diet as it is much harder to identify irritants and its longer more drawn out length makes it far more difficult to stick to.

10.6   Phase 1 – Full Elimination

In this diet, we start by eliminating all the major allergens, all complex carbohydrates and complex proteins, traditional "reflux foods", and all sugars and sweeteners. This is the quickest way to your baby being better, and especially useful they have lots of symptoms and constant digestive complaints regardless of what you eat. It is also the best diet if you are showing any digestive symptoms yourself.

If you know you or your baby to have an intolerance or allergy to anything in this suggest diet, then do not include those foods in your diet and substitute with something you know to be safe.

This is a very short term diet only, designed to support the reduction in symptoms for your baby, and then grow your food variety quickly again. We do not focus on nutritional elements in this stage, your body should have appropriate reserves of iron, calcium etc. Once we establish a "Place of Great" for baby, then we can look to reintroduce high nutritionally dense foods.

Your food list for this first phase is any of the following (as long as neither you nor your baby currently react to them).

Vegetables	Animal Produce	Fruit	Condiments
Asparagus	Chicken	Avocado	Honey
Beetroot	Lamb	Ripe Banana	Olive oil
Broccoli	Pork	Olives (*fresh only*,	Salt (I only
Cauliflower	Turkey	not preserved in	use Pink
Courgette		anything other	Himalayan
Cucumber		than oil or water)	Crystal Salt
Pumpkin			
Spinach			
Squashes (flesh only)			
– pumpkin, coquina,			
acorn, queen etc.			

There is always a risk that baby may react to some these foods, and if you observe any worsening with a food, you should stop consuming it immediately, wait until symptoms subside and replace it with another. This is because any person can react to any food, our body's are totally unique that way!

In fact there are no completely safe foods. This is the list most likely to be safe for your baby.

If your baby is on an acid blocking medication, pay attention to fats such as avocado as feeding these to baby direct may result in constipation or other symptoms.

One of my private clients has this to say about her experience of following this elimination and rebuild plan: it has "made me feel less bloated and nauseous and given me a clear idea of how to discover which foods I and my baby need to avoid. It has also given me many ideas and suggestions for better, alternative foods to eat which I'm confident will improve the overall health of my whole family.

As an example of what your first weeks food and meals could look like, here

10.6.1   WEEK 1 SAMPLE MENU

This menu is an example of combining the foods that are most safe. This is purely to get your baby to their Place of Great. See the recipes section for ideas on varying your flavours by means of cooking in this first week. Remember, this is a short-term way of eating to get you to a place where you can enjoy a much greater variety of food that your baby can tolerate.

We are going for BIG results FAST.

	Breakfast	Lunch	Dinner	Snack
Day 1	Avocado with Salt	Chicken or turkey salad	Lamb with squash and courgette	Bananas Olives
Day 2	Avocado with Salt	Chicken or turkey salad	Pork with cauliflower and squash	Bananas Olives
Day 3	Fauxgurt	Chicken or turkey salad	Lamb with squash and courgette	Bananas Olives
Day 4	Fauxgurt	Chicken or turkey salad	Pork with cauliflower, courgette and spinach	Bananas Olives
Day 5	Fauxgurt	Chicken or turkey salad	Lamb with squash and courgette	Bananas Olives
Day 6	Fauxgurt	Chicken or turkey salad	Pork with cauliflower, courgette and spinach	Bananas Olives
Day 7	Avocado with Salt	Chicken or turkey salad with *almonds*	Roast lamb with roast cauliflower & squash, beetroot and spinach	Bananas Olives

In salads, use mild salad leaves only in the beginning such as iceberg, cos, romaine, butterhead, green, red or oak leaf lettuce, little gem. Avoid peppery, hot or spicy leaves like rocket (arugula), lambs leaf, watercress, dandelion leaves, chrysanthemum greens, purslane.

Stay on this phase until your baby is in their Place of Great. This can be different for every baby and is in relation to where they have come from, but for a baby who suffers with constipation only having a painful bowel movement every 10 days, this could be passing a painless bowel movement every 3 or 4 days. For a baby who experiences sleep apnoea and snoring, this could be completely settled breathing or snoring with no sleep apnoea episodes. This will be very different from one family to the next and there is no right or wrong answer.

Once you are happy with your baby's improvement and you both have had at least 3 days consistently good or great, then it is time to start reintroducing foods to your diet.

After 7 days you should see significant improvement in your baby and be ready to start introducing new foods. This is now the basis of your personal Safe Diet. Every food you successfully introduce without flaring reflux or other symptoms will be added to this.

If there is no improvement at all, and you have been sticking to this diet, then you need to revisit what is causing your baby's reflux as it is likely not related to their food. Also consult with your GP again.

10.6.2   SIDE EFFECTS

One of the biggest side effects of this diet is fatigue and low energy. This is because unless you have been eating a ketogenic diet before now, your body is not used to using fat as an energy source. After a week or so, your body will adjust.

If you plan that you will have low energy, and that this is okay, then you should take it easy, with any luck your baby will be more rested and sleeping better too so that you will be able to get more rest also.

This is also one of the reasons that I do not call this a pure elimination diet, I want to rebuild your food variety so that you can have the energy to fully embrace life.

10.7   PHASE 2 – REINTRODUCTION OF FOODS

When reintroducing foods, it is important to only introduce one food at a time.

If you notice any symptoms in your own body (e.g. bloating or discomfort), then there is a higher risk of these foods having an impact on your baby. An impact may or may not be observed through breastmilk, but if no visible reaction is seen in your baby from breastmilk you may continue to eat it (if you are not uncomfortable yourself, e.g. harmless wind!).

You should make a note of this food that you reacted to it, to have a head-start awareness that this food may affect your baby the same way. This is because your baby's gut flora is almost a mirror image of yours, and so intolerances or inability to digest some foods may be observed. This is not guaranteed to happen, but it is good to have an awareness around foods.

Leave at least 3 days between food reintroduction in your diet. With some foods (e.g. dairy produce, higher allergens), it is safer to leave 4 days. For the basic foods, however, 2 days is usually sufficient.

If you observe any symptoms in your baby. Stop eating the recently introduced food, go back a few days to a diet you knew was safe until all of baby's symptoms resolve and then introduce another food. Do not try the food that was introduced and caused symptomatic reactions. Park this food for the moment, making note of it and the symptoms observed.

Refer to the list at the back of this book for the list of symptoms to be observant for. Any of these could be a reaction to a food.

10.7.1   FOODS TO INTRODUCE

Choosing foods from the following table to introduce to your diet, you should choose those food first that are going to add ease and pleasure to your life!

For example, if you succeed with eggs and ground almonds, this opens up the options of baking muffins as a snack for yourself! If you succeed with onions and garlic then you are good for the basis of soups, stir fry's etc.

I would recommend looking to trial eggs early as they are an amazingly nutritious food. Try egg yolks first, and then baked whole eggs if yolks prove ok. This way, if you get no symptoms or flare up with egg yolk, but you do with baked eggs, you can safely determine it is the egg white that baby has reacted to.

Vegetables	Animal Produce	Fruit	Other foods
Bell peppers Broccoli Cabbages (savoy, kale, nero, chard, red) Carrot Celery Kohlrabi Garlic Leeks Marrow Onion Purple Sprouting Romanesco	Egg yolks Egg whites (baked) Egg whites (lightly cooked) Continental Hams (Parma, prosciutto – hams that are just pork & salt) Bacon (minimise additives) Salmon Mackerel Cod Fish other than tuna	Coconut Mango Papaya Pineapple Grapes Lemons Limes Oranges Raspberries Tomato flesh (Passata or puree) Plums	Coconut oil (aroma free / odourless) Ground Nuts – e.g. Ground Almonds Nut Butters (almond butter, cashew, hazelnut – all smooth without skins) Pepper Herbs (bay, parsley, chives, tarragon, oregano, dill, marjoram, sage, rosemary) Spices (not hot – for flavour, e.g. turmeric, cumin, paprika, ginger, cinnamon, cloves, nutmeg) Cocoa Cacao Rude Health Almond Drink, Almond Milk, Hazelnut Milk and Coconut milk.

			Seeds:
			Quinoa
			Sesame (including tahini)
			Sunflower
			Pumpkin
			Coconut milk and cream (100% pure coconut)
			Herbal teas

Make a plan of the foods and drinks you would like to introduce and then stick to it.

If you know you and your baby are safe with dairy produce, you may also have milk produce, bovine, sheep and goat – milk, cream, cheese, yogurt, butter, ghee.

10.7.2   COMPLEX FOODS FOR MUM ONLY

There are some foods that mum might be able to digest fully and so the molecular level of the foods that pass to your baby through breastmilk is fully digested and won't cause your baby a problem. These foods will be individual to you and your baby, and so careful introduction should be taken with these. These foods are not suitable for your baby at this stage.

Vegetables	Animal Produce	Fruit	Other foods
White potatoes (peeled and pre-soaked only)	None	Very ripe pears (soft)	Rice (preferably organic white rice)
Sweet potatoes (peeled and pre-soaked only)		Very ripe melon (melons should have no green on the skin and be soft to touch when ripe)	Some legumes: garden peas, marrowfat peas, Red lentil pasta, sweetcorn (preferably frozen as not then stored in any additional preservatives)
		Seedy fruits – kiwi, whole RIPE tomatoes, strawberries, blueberries, pomegranate seeds	

10.7.3   FOODS TO AVOID COMPLETELY

In some foods, there are molecular level sugars and proteins that can pass into breastmilk from your blood. Some of these sugars may ferment in baby's gut because of the natural development of their digestive system and the limited digestive enzymes they have.

Vegetables	Animal Produce	Fruit	Other foods
White potatoes Sweet potatoes Parsnips Turnip Swede	Beef and Veal (if there is a known or suspected diary intolerance) All dairy produce – milk, cream, cheese, butter, ghee, yogurt All other milk produce – lactose free milk (unless you know this is safe), goats milk produce – milk, cream, cheese, yogurt, butter	Hard fruit – apples, pears, melon (we rarely if at all, get these "ripe") Dried fruit as sugars are too condensed	Legumes of all types including peas, beans, lentils, chickpeas, peanuts All Grains – either whole or processed, in any form Wheat, oats, rice, rye, barley, spelt, amaranth, millet etc. Alcohol (the sugars are too complex for baby's digestive system) Beef gelatin products (e.g. marshmallows) Sweeteners: Sugar, Agave, Maple syrup & sugar, sweet freedom, xylitol, artificial sweeteners, coconut sugar Vinegars

10.8   SAMPLE 28-DAY MEAL PLAN

The table over the next few pages is a suggested meal plan of how you could start this diet and then show you how to rebuild your foods, gradually and safely.

As you go through this process it is often about varying your food and diet. This is important to me, and so I have also created a recipe book alongside these foods that you can download from https://www.thebabyrefluxlady.co.uk/book-reader for free.

	Breakfast	Lunch	Dinner	Snack
Day 1	Avocado with Salt	Chicken or turkey salad	Lamb with squash and courgette	Bananas Olives
Day 2	Avocado with Salt	Chicken or turkey salad	Pork with cauliflower and squash	Bananas Olives
Day 3	Fauxgurt	Chicken or turkey salad	Lamb with squash and courgette	Bananas Olives
Day 4	Fauxgurt	Chicken or turkey salad	Pork with cauliflower, courgette and spinach	Bananas Olives
Day 5	Fauxgurt	Chicken or turkey salad	Lamb with squash and courgette	Bananas Olives
Day 6	Fauxgurt	Chicken or turkey salad	Pork with cauliflower, courgette and spinach	Bananas Olives
Day 7	Avocado with Salt	Chicken or turkey salad with *almonds*	Roast lamb with roast cauliflower & squash, beetroot and spinach	Bananas Olives
Day 8	Avocado with Salt	Chicken or turkey salad with almonds	Lamb with squash and courgette	Bananas Olives
Day 9	Avocado with Salt	Chicken or turkey salad *without almonds*	Pork with cauliflower and squash	Bananas Olives
Day 10	Fauxgurt	Chicken or turkey salad without almonds	Lamb with squash and courgette	Bananas Olives
Day 11	Fauxgurt	Chicken or turkey salad	Pork with cauliflower, courgette and *mushrooms*	Bananas Olives

Day 12	Fauxgurt	Chicken or turkey salad	Lamb with squash and courgette and mushrooms	Bananas Olives Almonds[126]
Day 13	Fauxgurt	Chicken or turkey salad	Pork with cauliflower, courgette and spinach	Bananas Olives Almonds
Day 14	Baked avocado with *egg*	Chicken or turkey salad	Roast lamb with roast cauliflower & squash, beetroot and spinach	Bananas Olives Almonds
Day 15	Baked avocado with egg	Chicken or turkey salad	Lamb with Squash and Courgette	Bananas Olives Almonds
Day 16	Banana slices with almond butter	Chicken or turkey salad	Pork with cauliflower, spinach and mushrooms	Bananas Olives Almonds
Day 17	Fauxgurt with *honey*	Chicken or turkey salad	Lamb with squash and courgette and mushrooms	Bananas Olives Almonds
Day 18	Baked avocado with egg	Chicken or turkey salad	Pork with cauliflower, courgette and spinach	Bananas Olives Almonds
Day 19	*Scrambled egg*	Chicken or turkey salad	Lamb with squash and courgette	Bananas Olives Almonds Banana muffins
Day 20	Banana slices with almond butter	Chicken or turkey salad	Pork with cauliflower, courgette and spinach	Bananas Olives Almonds Banana muffins

---

126 Add almonds as a snack as long as they have been deemed safe. If the whole nut has passed, then you can also include pure almond butter and ground almonds in your safe foods. Ground almonds can be used to "thicken" a vegetable mash and add some more bulk and consistency. our salads, and have a snack of banana with almond butter

Day 21	Banana slices with almond butter	Chicken or turkey salad	Cauliflower egg fried rice with mushrooms, broccoli & *peas*	Bananas Olives Almonds Banana muffins
Day 22	Avocado with Salt	Chicken or turkey salad	Cauliflower egg fried rice with mushrooms, broccoli & peas	Bananas Olives Almonds Banana muffins
Day 23	Scrambled egg with avocado	Chicken or turkey salad	Pork with broccoli and squash	Bananas Olives Almonds Banana muffins
Day 24	Fauxgurt	Chicken or turkey salad with *quinoa*	Lamb with Squash and Courgette	Bananas Olives Almonds Banana muffins
Day 25	Fauxgurt	Chicken or turkey salad with quinoa	Pork with cauliflower, courgette and mushrooms	Bananas Olives Almonds Banana muffins
Day 26	Baked avocado with egg	Chicken or turkey salad	Lamb with squash and beetroot	Bananas Olives Almonds Banana muffins
Day 27	***Chocolate avocado mousse***	Chicken or turkey salad	Pork with cauliflower, courgette and spinach	Bananas Olives Almonds Banana muffins
Day 28	Banana slices with almond butter	Chicken or turkey salad	Roast Lamb with Roast Cauliflower & Squash, Beetroot and Spinach	Bananas Olives Almonds Banana muffins

11 INTRODUCING SOLID FOOD

11.1   STARTING SOLIDS: MY STORY

When it came to weaning Sunflower, I attended a weaning workshop run by the local medical practice by the health visiting team. I was hoping to find out what I should feed my baby to give her the best start in life, help her learn to eat, and a bit about baby-appropriate portion sizes. What I actually got left me feeling shocked, scared and alone.

At this stage, I had only just found out about Sunflower's silent reflux. Sleep was a constant battle. Life was a constant battle! I was hoping – desperately hoping – for someone somewhere to tell me how to help my little bubba sleep. I was told in no uncertain terms by the health visiting team that day that – at 5 months – baby was old enough to be sleeping through the night. And if I had to leave her cry it out, that's what I should do. Thankfully, I trusted myself and knew Sunflower wasn't testing me each night just for kicks. She was in pain and I was her comfort.

The sentence that threw me, though, was this: "You should not feed your baby whole grains, or 'whole foods'. She can't digest it. She can have white bread, white pasta and white flour products instead."

Why would I feed my baby something I **know** to be devoid of any nutritional value, I wondered.

For years, we've been told to avoid "white" foods, they are so highly processed that they are equivalent to sugar with little or no nutritional value. In that meeting, I couldn't understand why would I feed my precious baby food that is not good for her. Why would I start putting her body through spikes and crashes from the first bites of food she eats? The health visitor couldn't answer. I asked what else I could feed her instead of these foods and she couldn't answer. I asked for the nutritional requirements of a 6-month-old and she couldn't answer me that either. All I got from her? "These are the NHS guidelines."

Media, healthcare, and every dietician and nutritionist on the planet have been insisting that white products like flour and rice are very high on the GI scale. They cause insulin to peak. We're also told they are low on the nutritional value scale compared to their whole grain counterparts. And here I was being told to feed these foods to my baby. The most precious thing in my life. I was confused. I couldn't marry the two. I wanted to give my baby the best start in life. How could I bring myself to feed her type-II-diabetes-causing foods? As a primary part of her diet?

I left that session feeling despair and horror in equal measure. Despair that I would have to continue to figure it out on my own and that this was the common information being given to every weaning parent. Horror that I had been given, in one sentence, the answer to why British children are some of the most obese in the world[127].

Armed with a few baby cookbooks and my own life-changing lifestyle transformation over the previous 5 years, I started deciding what I would make for Sunflower to eat. If I was going to do this on my own, it would be as good as I could make it.

As a believer that infancy provides the greatest opportunity for laying the foundations for a lifetime of strong health, I knew there were some foods I would not choose to feed my daughter. If a food was not good enough for me, it would not be good enough for Sunflower. Immediately, this ruled out wheat, gluten and refined sugars. I had already cut out dairy from my diet while breastfeeding and found some improvement in her symptoms. Yet with the start of solids, any improvement I might have seen on that front would go totally out the window.

---

127 When starting school, 23% of children in England were overweight or obese in 2015/2016. Data from State of Child Health, 2017, Royal College of Paediatrics and Child Health
https://www.rcpch.ac.uk/system/files/protected/page/SoCH%202017%20UK%20web%20updated.pdf

When I started teaching Sunflower how to eat, I did not have the appreciation for how a baby's digestive system worked like I do now. This was going to be a massive learning curve for us both.

I started baby with porridge oats. Not normal shop-bought-sugar-loaded-over-processed porridge, but organic jumbo oats, pre-soaked for 12 hours to make them more easily digestible for her. This is how I had my porridge so I just started giving Sunflower the same breakfast as me. She didn't take to it, so I thought to try some stewed fruit instead.

I loved a stewed apple, and since apple is on the common list of first baby foods[128], I thought this would be a good idea. Stewed apple was a hit. Seriously, Sunflower couldn't get enough of it. She gobbled it down eagerly. When the first small bowl was empty, she screamed at me for more! When I gave her a little more, she showed me her "I am loving this" excited happy face.

For her first meal of stewed apple, she ate a surprising amount. But when that bowl was empty, immediate screaming. She continued to scream for more when there was no more to have. She screamed at me for a solid 10 minutes until I gave in and gave her another milk feed, which settled her for a bit.

All the recommendations said to give a milk feed first, which I had done. The idea is that baby doesn't over-eat and still gets the necessary calories from milk. However, the only thing that would stop the screaming and settle her was stewed apple or boob. I was out of apple and thought she really had eaten enough, so I gave her boob.

This continued for days, maybe weeks. I introduced stewed apple, stewed pear. I mixed the fruit with porridge and she would eat it, so she was getting some oats, quinoa and other foods for breakfast.

---

128 https://www.nhs.uk/start4life/choosing-first-foods

The problem was Sunflower was more unsettled than ever. Her silent reflux was worse. Her sleeping was worse. She was straining for poos or not passing stools. Her tummy was constantly massively bloated. Neither of us was sleeping at night. I was barely surviving.

By this stage, I had given up my evenings in favour of sleeping beside her cot, which was set up like a nest bed beside mine. I dreaded the approach of 7pm every evening. I knew it was the start of a long night, though I always hoped it would be different tonight.

I couldn't bear constant waking in the middle of the night, because it would take us ages to get back to sleep. Typically, there were 90 minutes between Sunflower going to sleep and waking. Each time, it took my brain another hour to switch off, so I was averaging about 30 minutes of sleep every 2 hours. Exhaustion was not the word...

I was approaching depression, but I couldn't give in to the failure I perceived that to be. When 7am rolled around, I would get up and start the day as if I had the energy of a sleeping 2-year old. I kept going. I pushed and pushed. I shielded my true emotions from the world, including from my husband. I hid what I was feeling and desperately wanted to get to a better place for me and my daughter. I was desperate for help. Desperate to know what my daughter could eat without causing her so much distress. I was 100% convinced it was food, but I couldn't piece it together.

Then in August 2013, after 6 months of barely living, I had an experience where I finally felt understood. I met with two old friends, both of whom had daughters with cow's milk protein allergy. In both cases, the allergy was so severe that their daughters were at risk from anaphylaxis because of dairy. For the first time, I was speaking to other mums who genuinely believed me about the total lack of sleep and distress I was suffering.

They absolutely *knew* I wasn't exaggerating about our experience. They were mums who knew I couldn't leave my baby down. Mums who could identify with the struggles. Mums who, over dinner, both told me in no uncertain terms that I must *demand* to see a paediatric allergist for dairy allergy test. They were convinced this could be the magic bullet for us. Meeting these friends again was *so* important for my personal sanity and wellbeing at the time; simply talking to mums who believed me was an incredible unburdening, an enormous relief.

Back at home, I found a paediatric allergist, organised a referral. My GP thought I didn't need to see one, but I fought to get him to write a referral letter on the basis that I would see the allergist privately and wouldn't need the NHS to fund it. I went as soon as I could.

On first meeting, the allergist was a pleasant man, who empathised with an exhausted mum. We did the skin prick test. It came back negative. Sunflower had no allergies. On one hand, this was a relief. But on the other hand, what now? If she was not allergic to foods, what the hell was going on? He confirmed reflux and gave me a prescription for ranitidine. He looked at me as he said confidently, "I guarantee you'll phone me next week thanking me for changing your life". ***What cocky arrogance!***

I was finally starting to understand that my daughter was perfectly healthy. That reflux is a normal part of digestive development, but can be aggravated in some babies more than others. Sunflower's body was sensitive to foods that were not fit for babies to consume. She was teaching me a lot about food, development and the human body.

Over the previous 5 years, I had completely changed my own health and lifestyle. I came to understand how food interacted with my body, the chemistry. What I was missing was the knowledge of a baby's digestive system. Sunflower's digestive system was still immature, so I had to figure out what was best for her at what stage in her development.

With an allergy ruled out and still completely desperate, I turned to what I knew best. Analysis. It's what I was trained to do in my engineering career and it's what I did with engineering, maths and project management for 14 years in business. I knew there must be something going on with food because we'd had a few "better" nights. I just so far hadn't figured out what made for a good night or a bad night. I had tried all sorts of diets in vain. It was time to gather some data and search for the patterns.

I started a food and symptom diary for myself and Sunflower, and I did the greatest elimination diet ever. At the beginning, all I was eating and drinking was water, butternut squash, avocado and broccoli, so that was all I gave Sunflower too.

I did this for about a week and the change in Sunflower was remarkable. Night wakings had gone from 90 minutes screaming in agony to 5 minutes nuzzling and settling down again; she went from 8 or more times awake every night to 4 or 5 times awake. I didn't sleep much more initially – I kept waking up and needing to check that Sunflower was alive and breathing! But this was a welcome change, every time I went back to sleep smiling to myself.

Gradually, we introduced new foods and by 9 months we had her reflux under control. Sunflower was a year old when her reflux disappeared completely. She had a varied diet, we manged to create a tasty chocolate birthday cake for her and life was getting so much better.

Introducing food is a balancing act, because you want to introduce flavours as much as possible before baby develops an awareness to "turn up their nose" at food and throw it back at you! You need tactics for managing the "fussy eater". Pick foods from the list that are highly dense from a nutritional standpoint and low on the allergy/intolerance response list. Giving your child a wide range of tastes and options early in life will develop their palate, and give them the opportunity to explore eating and tasting. This is a gift for life.

The next big step in baby's digestive maturity is the ability to digest food that is anything other than milk. Babies with food intolerances or allergies are particularly sensitive to the food they eat. Other parents and I found that reflux is often under control by the time it comes to solids, and then symptoms reappear with a vengeance, so mums find themselves tearing their hair out again, wondering what has gone wrong so suddenly. In fact, 54% of babies appear to relapse with food.

11.2   Weaning/Complementary Feeding

Weaning is the term most commonly used to indicate that baby is starting to eat solids. Confusion often arises as it also means the beginning of the end of breastfeeding. In fact, starting to eat solids does not mean the end of breastfeeding at all, the two are mutually exclusive.

We often forget about everything baby's body needs to be able to do before feeding solid food. We also can be confused about how to balance milk and food. This certainly confused me immediately: "Am I supposed to feed baby less milk straight away?" Some of the food was going in but I wasn't sure how much went on the bib, face, arms, highchair, floor and me! So tricky.

So with all that in mind, we have complementary feeding. Complementary feeding is just what the title says – ***complementary***. It is not designed to sustain baby, but to introduce your wee one to food and start the digestive system working. Milk continues to be the *primary* source of energy past 6 months of age. The saying "food before 1 is just for fun" holds some truth.

From 6 months to 2 years, baby's digestive system and nutritional requirements do not change massively from what they were at 3 months. Baby is designed to get most their calorific intake to fuel brain development (the fastest and most demanding part of infant development).

As I've explained, it makes sense that complementary feeding follows a similar pattern of 55:39:6 fat to sugars to protein calorific breakdown, until baby has developed teeth and a capacity to produce enzymes.

11.3   INTRODUCING FOOD

Foods should be introduced to your baby in a gentle and slow manner, *one food at a time with 4 days between new foods*.

Your baby must learn how to eat. You baby is experiencing new textures and tastes, experimenting with the feelings of eating and swallowing food, not just liquid. There is a lot for a developing baby to cope with.

I recommend the following guidelines for introducing food, which we will look at in more detail in the coming sections:

1. Make sure baby is ready
2. Establish a positive eating environment
3. Start from a Place of Great
4. Understand your baby's symptoms
5. Take your time
6. Remove your assumptions
7. Ignore "meal rules"
8. Have fun
9. Trust your baby and follow their lead supportively
10. Eat with your baby
11. Exaggerate the movements you want your baby to learn
12. Watch out for any signs of discomfort
13. Observe and record.

11.3.1   MAKE SURE BABY IS READY

Parents of reflux-y babies are commonly advised to introduce solids early in a hope that the new thickness of the stomach contents will help the food stay in the stomach and reduce reflux. I disagree with this advice. It is illogical to my mind to introduce solid foods before baby is physiologically ready for solid foods. It's like telling a parent to give their child a sharp knife and they will learn to cut! Some will, but many will hurt themselves in the process.

In line with standard guidelines, before introducing solids, baby should be able to:

- Sit upright on their own and hold head steady
- Co-ordinate eyes, hands and mouth, meaning they can pick up the food and get it into their mouth by themselves (not necessarily with a spoon!)
- Swallow food. If baby pushes the food back out with the tongue, they are not yet ready to start on solids.

These are physical signs that baby's body is now mature enough to *start* digesting solid foods.

There are many opinions on spoon-feeding or baby-led-weaning. There are pros and cons to both. You can even combine the two! I recommend doing what feels right for you and your family. Take time to do a little research and find out what works for you. With my first child, I was so in-control that it was spoon all the way. With my second, she was sitting on my lap at dinner time one evening and I saw her helping herself to squash chips from my plate! Guess she was ready then! Clearly, that time around, it was more baby-led, but plenty of spoon-fed meals when I needed the convenience of a quick tidy-up and timely mealtime. See what suits you and don't be afraid to mix it up!

11.3.2   Establish A Positive Eating Environment

Remember, babies have the greatest opportunity to experiment and trial foods available to them during infancy. They have virgin taste buds, and can eat and taste everything in the world with zero preconceptions of what it will taste like. Do not limit your baby's tastes and nutritional intake potential with your own eating patterns.

11.3.3   Start From A Place of Great

The aim is to get your baby to the happiest most settled place before you start to introduce solids. For many babies, their Place of Great will not be perfect, or even great. That is okay. Do everything you can to make sure baby is well-rested before introducing food, so that lack of sleep is not an excuse.

11.3.4   UNDERSTAND BABY'S SYMPTOMS

It is important to understand and document how your baby is doing right from the start. You must understand and record all the symptoms they have, so you can observe changes. Like getting your baby to a Place of Great, if you understand what their symptoms are on their best day, then you can use this as the baseline to monitor ups and downs.

11.3.5   TAKE YOUR TIME

With baby having nothing but milk for 6 months, remember that a bit of avocado is fabulous variety. It represents 50% change! The day your baby turns 6 months is not the day to flip a switch to "eats everything" mode.

If there is going to be any reaction (allergic or intolerance response), it could take up to 4 days to manifest. Hence, the recommendation of one food at a time every 4 days ensures there are no delayed reactions "pending" that could then be wrongly interpreted as a reaction to a more recently introduced food.

11.3.6   REMOVE YOUR ASSUMPTIONS

Remove your own preconceptions of food from the equation. Take everything you know about food and throw it out the window. You have probably been eating and consuming for well over 20 years, maybe a lot more, maybe a bit less. For now, your eating habits should not inform how you feed your infant.

There will come a time in your child's future when your choices around food can most definitely influence their meals. But at the start, be patient with them. Put yourself in their shoes. Imagine what it is like to be bombarded every day with new sensory experiences.

Food, for your baby, is many multiple new things among many multiple new things. Food awakens the taste buds, has different textures, different temperatures. There are so many varieties!

If your husband, partner, mother-in-law, sister or any other interested party advises differently, ask them to kindly shut up and butt out. You might hear, "Give baby everything from your plate". No. Your baby's needs are your baby's needs. You are taking care, taking your time. The reward will come from a slow and gentle approach, because any reflux flare-ups will be minimised or not present at all, potential irritants avoided, and baby will get the most from their food, all while sleeping better and being happier.

If it's your partner who objects, ask them to read this book first. If they appear unsupportive of your choice, it's time for an honest conversation. You need their support in this, and so does your child. You both want what's best for your baby. You both want to get back to a place where your relationship is no longer overshadowed by reflux, right? You both want to get back to a place where life is much easier than it has been since baby arrived, don't you? This is a massive step in that direction.

11.3.7   IGNORE "MEAL RULES"

Culturally, we have come to accept a number of foods as being more or less suitable for breakfast, lunch, dinner, tea and supper. In truth, these definitions are futile. What is needed is a balanced approach to food **_overall_**.

If your baby wants to eat avocado dipped in egg yolk and smothered in olive oil for breakfast, that is fine! Apart from the crazy amount of brain-building fats consumed, later in the day or week they may choose to have nothing but a massive portion of butternut squash for dinner or a head of broccoli straight from the supermarket trolley (this has happened!) There is no way we can balance an infant's meals perfectly at every sitting. A better goal is to balance the meals over a week.

11.3.8   HAVE FUN

From 6 months, baby is ready to start to _learn_ how to eat. Not ready _to_ eat. These are subtly different. We should recognise and respect that.

The day you see your baby sitting up on their own and holding their head steady, and you know they have reasonable hand-eye coordination, is not the day they start eating full meals. Until this point, it's only been suckling and swallowing on the part of the mouth. Baby should be expressing an interest in putting food (and possibly everything else!) into their mouth. If the tongue reflex pushes food back out immediately, they are not ready to learn how to eat and need to learn a bit more about their mouth first.

You can give baby food to play with. This is all part of the food game. You can make meal times fun and engaging. If you are worried about what you are feeding your little one, if you are worried about pain in the belly all night from this meal or that, baby will pick up on these stresses.

Having a plan, taking it slowly and gently will give you the confidence that your baby's meals are good for them to digest and reassurance that they'll have a good day and night. You can relax and enjoy the fun of food together.

11.3.9   LET BABY LEAD

Let your baby lead in the amount of food they choose to eat. Do not force them to eat more. Not only is baby learning how to eat, but also about textures, tastes and temperature too. This is a new process to your little one and they may want to take their time with it. All babies are different and learn at different paces and in different styles. Give them the respect to learn their way.

If you choose to spoon-feed your baby, do not force baby to eat and swallow. If food comes back out of the mouth, that is fine. Let your baby lead and you follow. This is their time to learn. Trust what their body is telling them.

11.3.10   EAT WITH YOUR BABY

There are some important aspects of eating around your baby. Your baby will learn from you and siblings first and foremost.

If you offer everything in a non-judgemental manner, baby will likely accept it in that way. If you are willing to taste food, baby will likely be willing to taste food too. If you turn your nose up at broccoli, your child will "learn" that they don't like broccoli without ever even trying it. Even if baby starts out eating everything, as a toddler, they will learn your food aversions and dislikes without recognition of the food that's actually in their mouth, regardless of their own taste buds.

Therefore, it's a really, *really*, **really** important part of making sure your child has the best and correct balance of nutrition and food to be the best teacher you can be. I know a mum (or three!) who "detests" vegetables. These mums were simply amazing when it came to weaning their children and recognised that it would be unhealthy for their kids to have the same dislikes of vegetables as they did. They spent **hours** lovingly cooking and preparing fabulous healthy meals for their babies. Fast-forward 5 years and these children now refuse to eat anything that is considered to be a vegetable. Their diet is primarily sausages, fish fingers, chicken nuggets, chips and beans.

Now, I'm not a complete no on foods like these for kids, but I do think they should be having more vegetables. (Did you spot the colour green in their food?) Also, I would suggest vegetables without sugar added. I am sad to say that, despite parents' heroic efforts to **provide** healthy foods, babies' behaviour will always be overridden by the observation of their parents' actions.

Children are much more likely to **do what you do**, rather than what you say, so be aware!

11.3.11   EXAGGERATE WHAT BABY NEEDS TO LEARN

We take for granted that our babies will eat. We tend to forget just how much activity must be done to eat. As adults, we don't need to think about eating. We put something in our mouth. We decide if it is food or not. If it is, we figure out if it needs chewing. If it does, we chew. We chew to a point of knowing we can swallow safely. These activities are unconscious activities, because we have done them so many times that our muscles know what to do.

For most us, walking is the same. When it comes to walking, we understand and observe how baby needs to think about it and consciously learn what to do before they no longer have to think about it anymore. The same can be said for eating. We must teach our children how to eat. And teach them to eat even better than we do ourselves. They're not yet producing pancreatic enzymes, so mixing salivary amylase well with their carbohydrates is all-important for better digestion of those foods and less irritation to the digestive system.

The greatest skill you can teach your child with eating is *chewing*. Chewing mushes the food. Chewing stimulates the secretion of saliva (and so, amylase). Chewing mixes the food with the saliva to start the digestive process. The longer your baby chews food, the more saliva will be mixed through.

Getting your baby to imitate the chewing action is the best teaching you can provide. Babies and children copy what they observe, so make sure you're showing them this yourself.

11.3.12   SIGNS OF DISCOMFORT

Observing and reading your baby when introducing food is especially important. Do not expect it all to go swimmingly in the first meal. Your baby has much to learn.

Signs of discomfort to look out for when introducing foods to your reflux baby are:

1. Crying between spoonfuls
2. Acting like they cannot get enough, especially when you think they have had loads
3. Excessive excitement about food
4. Excessive crying after a meal soothed only by milk
5. Stretching their head or neck upwards
6. Arching in their chair, like they might be fighting against the straps
7. Hiccoughs
8. Rash
9. Hives
10. Wheezing

11. Other symptoms listed in section 3.1 Symptoms: What To Look For (page 30).

Signs 1-6 are signs that could be interpreted as "baby loves their food". However, in a reflux baby, they are more often a sign that the particular food is causing pain or discomfort. If your baby has reflux, it may be that their oesophagus is raw from the acid regurgitating from the stomach. If this is the case, some foods will cause further irritation and burning on raw skin. Any time you observe these behaviours, stop feeding that food *immediately*. Offer baby milk, as this often soothes the burning. Give baby a day or so to recover and try a different food.

If your baby is suffering with any pain whatsoever when eating, do not force them to eat. This could cause a food aversion. Rather, take it slowly at this stage and be led by them.

Hiccoughs are a sign that your baby is eating too fast as they have gulped air. Hiccoughs are an effective way of the body getting rid of excess air[129], so there is no need to try and stop them unless your baby is decidedly uncomfortable.

11.3.13   Purées or Lumps?

I love baby-led weaning (BLW) for its simplicity, just as I love purées for their convenience. (Freezer food, anyone?) That said, BLW is not always a suitable as a gentle approach for babies with immature and sensitive digestive systems, for the following reasons.

When it comes to carbohydrates and proteins, I prefer to start with purees. Lumps and chunks are better suited to the fat-source foods. To explain why, allow me a quick recap.

As we know, your baby only produces amylase for digesting starches and sugars in the mouth. When they start eating, babies do not know how

---

129 Howes, D. (2012). Hiccups: A new explanation for the mysterious reflex. Bioessays, 34(6), 451–453. https://www.ncbi.nlm.nih.gov/pmc/articles/PMC3504071/

to chew. Chewing is so important because it physically mashes the food as well as mixing the food with saliva. That said, most of us chew too little and swallow lumpy food. This is okay for adult digestive systems where we have stronger stomach acid and plenty of pancreatic activity to support ongoing digestion. In your baby's body, saliva contains the only sugar enzyme they have, so the more mixing of food they can do in their mouth, the better the digestion of the food.

By giving your baby purees and encouraging them to "play" with the food in their mouths, they will increase their exposure of food to salivary amylase to support digestion throughout the digestive tract. Add breastmilk into vegetables too, because it has its own amylase included to support infant digestion.

Mix proteins with ripe tropical fruit that have their own digestive enzymes[130]. The natural digestive enzymes in these fruits can support the breakdown of proteins. You may observe irritation of a protein on its own, but when combining the food with a ripe tropical fruit, that it is much better tolerated. Now you know the reason!

Fats are a different matter. Infants have a relatively higher capability for fat digestion in the stomach than adults[131]. The churning action of the stomach will be able to cope with small lumps swallowed in bitten-off chunks. Foods like egg yolk and avocado can be given in lumps. Take care with egg yolks to break them into smaller chunks from the round before offering it to your baby.

11.3.14   DO'S AND DON'TS FOR FEEDING YOUR BABY
Do

- Give baby a full milk feed just before solids
- Encourage chewing and eating

---

130 http://www.alive.com/health/the-juicy-story-on-tropical-fruit/
131 https://www.ncbi.nlm.nih.gov/pmc/articles/PMC370635/

- Make yourself laugh at how silly you feel with exaggerated mouth movements
- Eat the same food as your baby, with your baby
- Let your baby try to feed you if interested
- Encourage positive playful fun at all stages
- Eat outside or cover the floor with a paper table cloth that you can easily clean
- Make meal times fun
- Encourage your baby to drink water
- Make enough to store for a few days in the fridge so you can reduce prep time
- Have your camera at the ready for Food Face photos! Especially important for a working parent!
- Keep a food and symptom diary for this next few weeks
- Show your baby that you enjoy the food, regardless of whether you do or not. Your facial expressions when it comes to food are much more telling than your words and your baby is an excellent reader of you, whether you know it or not! Your baby will copy what you do much sooner than what you say!
- Introduce new foods in small portions. Give that food to baby on all 4 days (provided you have not witnessed any negative reactions), each day without reference or preconceptions from the day before.

Don't

- Get stressed about meal times, as your baby is extremely sensitive to your emotions
- Force baby to eat food. Remember how much they have to learn!
- Put out massive portions! Rather, little by little. If baby wants more, they can have more!
- Be worried if there is more food in baby's hair than in their mouth!
- Feel like you *have* to feed baby every day initially. If you forget, feel exhausted, are going out and it would be easier to just have milk, that's okay.

- Feel like you have to immediately jump to three solid meals per day. Again, respect how much baby is learning.
- Be afraid to try new things, but **do** make sure you do it with your food diary to hand
- Put your food aversions and judgements onto your baby's foods and meal times. Meaning... for your baby, food is an entirely new experience where repetition is key to learning and development success. At the first taste of a food, baby may make a face that you read as "dislike". However, this face could be saying, "What is this? It's a bit strange!" Your baby will need more exposure to the food and more time to try it until they can decide if they "like" it or not.
- Equally, don't force your baby to eat something they don't want. It may be that the first taste on the first day was a strange new texture them, and they don't want any more that day. Don't force them to eat more. Just introduce the food again tomorrow without preconceptions.

11.4   WHAT FOODS FIRST?

This is a really important question. You will have gathered by now that my approach is different to that of the standard approach to introducing food. And so, the foods that I suggest you introduce to your baby are very different too. I focus on three key things:

- Baby's ability to physically breakdown the food
- Nutritional value of the food
- Energy density

So the foods you should start with are those that are going to give you the greatest 'bang-for-buck'. Babies are designed to digest fats, so you should start there.

Remember, never give your baby a food you know they have an allergy to without proper supervision and guidance from your allergist.

The best first food in my opinion, is avocado. Ripe avocado. Actually all fruits should be fully ripe. Then foods like ripe banana, well-cooked egg yolk (if baby can tolerate eggs), olive oil. For the full list of the "safer" foods, refer to section 9.3 Safe Foods (page191).

If you really want to take the pain out of introducing food to your baby and make it as easy as possible on yourself, you can join my Reflux Free Baby e-course that gives you meal plans, recipes and much more content with bonus content being added all the time, because there is more to parenting than food! Visit http://geni.us/RefluxFreeBaby for more details.

PART 4

REFLUX
REPERCUSSIONS
& RELATIONSHIPS

12 Sleep For Unsettleable Babies & Parents

One of the biggest problems for parents of unhappy babies is sleep. Or I should say: a distinct lack of it. Sleep is under-rated until you're the parent of an unsettled baby, when you get a real understanding of how sleep deprivation works as a form of torture.

Your baby will find places and times to sleep, napping on a shoulder, in a car, on a walk, in a carrier. Sometimes, even during the night when baby is so physically exhausted from screaming all day that they sleep well at night. It might be that baby is not getting the amount of sleep they really need at this age, but their body can manage by grabbing 40 winks every time they feed, every time they are somewhere comfortable.

You, on the other hand, cannot just grab a snooze every few minutes. Even if you could, it doesn't work for your mind or body because you are no longer wired to function on anything less than 6 hours sleep, never mind nothing but broken sleep.

12.1   *YOUR* Sleep: Quality, Then Quantity

This chapter is about getting you and your baby better quality sleep as a priority, and then more of it. There are several tips and strategies that you can try to figure out what might work best for you.

One of the most challenging aspects of being the mum of a baby with reflux, silent reflux, colic or a food intolerance is that it often presents itself at night. Baby cannot lie down flat for any period of time, baby will only sleep in mum's arms, baby wakes after about 30-90 minutes of sleep. You are barely asleep before you're awake again.

The first thing to realise is that changing baby's sleep habits are reliant on (a) baby being able to sleep and being comfortable first, then (b) teaching baby night and day. These are not mutually exclusive (as I treated them in the early days). In fact, working on one at a time can help the whole family.

Almost every mother will experience a level of reduced sleep with a little baby, but for mums of babies with high needs, the period of sleep deprivation can run to months, or years.

While I believe we are, in part, able to deal with reduced sleep after having a baby, we should not expect ourselves to be able to function at our pre-child highest levels. Yet, this is what we and others demand of ourselves. We expect that having a baby should be an event that brings a child into our world and then lets us get on with life. Not true. Having a baby is a *major* life event. Expecting no changes in response to such an event is naïve.

This is about *you* now, Mum. I want to help *you* get better sleep. You may not have control over how much sleep you get, but I think you can take control of the *quality* of that sleep.

12.1.1   REASONS TO IMPROVE YOUR SLEEP

Sleep deprivation is a serious condition in itself. There are so many risks and problems caused by reduced sleep alone that it is a major area of research in our society. And lack of this shut-eye stuff has been scientifically proven to cause:

1. Difficulty in controlling emotional aspects:
    a. Mood swings
    b. Irrational behaviour
    c. Emotional outbursts
    d. Intense feelings of overwhelm
    e. Feelings of paranoia or delirium
    f. Impulsivity
2. Mental illness
    a. Stress
    b. Depression
    c. Anxiety

3. Physiological problems
    a. Reduced immunity
    b. Increased blood pressure
    c. Impaired blood glucose control
    d. Increased inflammation
    e. Overeating
    f. Weight gain
    g. Inability to lose weight
    h. Poor libido[132]
4. Reduced cognitive processes that reduce learning ability by impairing[133]:
    a. Attention
    b. Alertness
    c. Concentration
    d. Decision-making abilities
    e. Judgement
    f. Memory
    g. Problem-solving
    h. Reasoning

It is also strongly associated with increased risk of:

1. Obesity
2. Diabetes
3. High blood pressure
4. Heart disease
5. Reduced life expectancy
6. Heart attack
7. Stroke

That's a scary list. And I know I am in there too. Though I'm sort of happy there's a good reason I'm not losing any more weight, despite my efforts at the moment of writing this!

---

132 http://www.nhs.uk/Livewell/tiredness-and-fatigue/Pages/lack-of-sleep-health-risks.aspx
133 http://www.webmd.com/sleep-disorders/features/10-results-sleep-loss#1

Interestingly, sleep deprivation also impairs judgement, about everything, including sleep itself! "Studies show that over time, people who are getting six hours of sleep, instead of seven or eight, begin to feel that they've adapted to that sleep deprivation – they've gotten used to it," Gehrman says. "But if you look at how they actually do on tests of mental alertness and performance, they continue to go downhill. So there's a point in sleep deprivation when we lose touch with how impaired we are."[134]

The lack of sleep wreaks havoc on your internal body clock, which is vital in maintaining normal body processes. That's because sleep is a true "second state of being" with functions and processes of its own.

We all know that sleep can make us feel on top of the world and able to cope with anything life throws at us. Conversely, a single night of poor sleep can make the whole world come crashing down. We cannot cope with anything, are moody, eat badly, make awful decisions. That's because sleep is an essential physiological process for the sustainment of life.

Some of the responsibilities of good sleep are[135]:

1. To facilitate and organise long-term memory
2. To physically restore the body through tissue and cell restoration and repair
3. Neutralisation of neurotoxins
4. To restore normal levels of chemicals throughout our bodies
5. Strengthening of the immune system.

If you implement good sleep hygiene for yourself as well as your baby, you will both benefit. And with such a strong correlation between sleep deprivation and postnatal depression, you will be doing yourself and your baby a massive favour by supporting yourself. Look after yourself.

---

134 Phil Gehrman, PhD, assistant professor of psychiatry and clinical director, BehavioUral Sleep Medicine Program, University of Pennsylvania, Philadelphia

135 https://www.howsleepworks.com/why_restoration.html

Being a mum is challenging enough. With sleep as a further serious challenge, I hope to help you find some strategies that can get you and your baby a better night's rest.

If you can improve your quality of sleep, you will feel better. If you can then improve the quantity of sleep you get, fabulous!

A study in April 2016 concluded that "interventions designed to improve maternal sleep and postpartum mood should include both mothers and infants, because improving infant sleep alone is not likely to improve maternal sleep, and poor infant sleep is linked to postpartum depression and stress."[136]

12.2   BABY SLEEP ROUTINE

A good sleep routine is essential for baby and mum. Sleep is a massive area of research now, and studies show that a poor bedtime routine can directly cause obesity with all its associated health problems in adults[137]. As a mum, if you want to be at your best, as good as that looks for the moment with an unhappy baby, you'll need to establish a better bedtime routine.

You may think I'm being totally unreasonable. There is no such thing as a predictable when it comes to being able to go to bed early, get a good night's rest, or even to dream of such a thing! Every evening, all you can think is that dreaded: *What's this evening going to look like?*

But I'm here to tell you that your baby's unhappy tummy is probably predictable. It's predictable that you'll be up during the night walking around the house lulling baby to sleep, bouncing or doing squats, and

136 Sharkey, K. M., Iko, I. N., Machan, J. T., Thompson-Westra, J., & Pearlstein, T. B. (2016). Infant Sleep and Feeding Patterns are Associated with Maternal Sleep, Stress, and Depressed Mood in Women with a History of Major Depressive Disorder. Archives of Women's Mental Health, 19(2), 209–218. http://doi.org/10.1007/s00737-015-0557-5

137 Roenneberg T, Allebrandt KV, Merrow M, Vetter C. Social jetlag and obesity. Curr Biol. 2012 May 22;22(10):939-43. doi: 10.1016/j.cub.2012.03.038. Epub 2012 May 10. Erratum in: Curr Biol. 2013 Apr 22;23(8):737. PubMed PMID: 22578422.

getting beautiful legs in the process! There is predictability in the lack of sleep. There is predictability in the multiple wake-ups. You feel they're inevitable, right? So, don't fight them. Accept them. Accept all the things that are contributing to you being exhausted right now. And work with them, not against them.

I've got some tips to share from a time I was deeply familiar with exhaustion. This is what I learned when I was shattered with my first baby. And they led me to being not-so-shattered with my second.

Believe me when I say my second child had just as many night wakings, possibly more, even to this day. As I write this book, she is 3 years old and still waking every night. She has spent **one** night not in my bed and 2 without me in hers since she was born. And yet, I'm in a place mentally, emotionally and physically that I can run a business, function at a reasonably normal level, and not be bothered by the lack of sleep. In fact, we both sleep better knowing one is beside the other.

Why? How? Take a deep breath and let me explain...

12.2.1   NIGHT-TIME STRATEGIES

If you want anything to improve, you must first accept that you must change. Your behaviours, your expectations. Once you change these, *everything* becomes easier. And while the long-term goal is to get baby to a place where they're sleeping through the night like a happy little camper, that takes time. In the meantime, you have to do what you can. And there's *plenty* you can do.

Remember, a happy mum is a happier baby. Yes, it's a two-way street, and as mum, *you* must take the first step!

If you're anything like me, you would *finally* get baby out of your arms as it's time to make dinner. You'd sit down with your other half whom you haven't seen since morning, if he didn't leave the house before you actually saw him. Your only adult contact of the day is so precious that you cannot give it up and I'm not suggesting you do. Here's some thoughts on how to structure your evening a little differently, so you can get more quality in.

I used to breastfeed in front of the TV, camped on the sofa from 7:30pm until whenever I got to bed. Most nights, this was about 11pm. Normally, a few minutes before I planned on leaving the sofa, Sunflower would wake, get upset, need bouncing, rocking, winding, massage, infant drops, gripe water, or just more boob to help her with wind. I had about 3 hours of this. Every single night.

It became – you guessed it – **predictable**. And I gave up fighting it.

You should stop fighting it too. You can re-plan and restructure your evening with your partner so that you get time together **and** some sleep. What you think you're missing out on really isn't that important. You're not going to get them in your current routine... The latest episode of GoT will be available on catch up; you can read your book next week; you can phone your mum in the morning; your partner can help you with most of the suggestions here.

I suggest:

1. ***Spending a few days recording and understanding baby's symptoms and habits*** – these will form the basis of what your evening timings *should* look like. For example, is baby happy sleeping for 1-3 hours on you after a 7pm feed? Use this time to get rest for yourself too. When baby is up in the evening, is it 20 minutes or 3 hours to settle? Then how much longer to return to sleep?
   If you're like me, you already have all this information logged in a sleep timer app. If you're not, download my free food and symptom diary template (which also tracks sleep). Print out a few pages and complete them for 3 to 5 days to unveil your baby's natural evening routine.

   Don't waste your own time thinking, *I'll remember this in the morning.* If your night-time is long and disturbed, you won't remember any of it: how many times you woke, how you settled baby that time, if you snoozed or not, none of it.

2. ***Deciding on a bedtime routine for baby and sticking to it*** – having a strong bedtime routine already established for baby will help when their sleep does improve. Children up to the age of 5 need 11 to 12 hours of night-time sleep, so it makes sense to start a bedtime now that will suit you when it comes time for pre-school and school. I suggest sleep by 7-7:30pm, which gives you a wake up of 6:30-7:30am.

Of course, this will be different for a young baby, because at birth your baby doesn't know day from night, except that day is night and night is day! Implementing a routine early will start to set the foundation for good sleepers later, even if it doesn't feel like it now. Additionally, a good night-time routine for your own wellbeing is a must.

3. ***Work back from a target sleep time of 7:30pm*** – and don't worry about where or how baby goes to sleep. If baby's evening feed is going to take an hour, then you need to have had your dinner and be ready to go to bed too. Bath at 6:00pm, baby massage at 6:20pm, into the sleep environment for 6:30pm for bedtime feed.

You know what? I know that this feels like a lot of planning, a lot of constraints and a lot of "things to get done when I don't want to do them". Take it from a former impulsive live-life-by-the-seat-of-my-pants person that this is the start of getting your life back! It starts with self-care. Sleep is the most important self-care activity you can do. It is ***way*** more important than even a shower!

So, by 6:30pm you and your baby are nursing/feeding, maybe in a chair or in your bed, in a darkened room. This starts to show that there is a difference between night and day, and that it's signalled by darkness.

12.3   SLEEP ENVIRONMENT

The sleep environment is incredibly important; not just for teaching baby the difference between night and day, but for achieving a higher *quality* of sleep for parents.

In January 2015, Sunflower (now 2) was in and out of our bedroom *loads*. We were being woken up *and* were unable to get back to sleep quickly. Her night wakings had become so disruptive that we needed to figure out how to get better *quality* sleep rather than simply more of it. This prompted my better half, J, to start some research.

What he discovered changed our lives!

12.3.1   Light

Light from the blue spectrum suppresses the secretion of melatonin – our sleep hormone, and this blue light is in daylight. In the absence of daylight, our brains produce melatonin and we feel sleepy. There are two prerequisites for the production of melatonin – darkness and your personal night-time.

Yes, *your* night-time – linked to *your* circadian rhythm, *your* 24-hour body clock. If you sleep during the day, your body will not produce melatonin, so going into a restful deep sleep is less likely. Some people, such as night-workers, can alter their body's personal night-time through careful practice, but as a mum, this doesn't work. You are wiser to recognise that night-time is when it is dark outside!

Life has evolved such that few of us wake and sleep with the sun. It's not practical in our modern culture. Imagine sleeping from 5pm til 8am in the winter (bliss!) and then only from 10pm til 4am in the summer (erm... not so bliss). Winter days may not be as productive.

It is now the norm for us to be awake well past the first hours of darkness at night. When this first started being the case, people used candlelight, which doesn't emit blue light; hence, they did not suffer with melatonin disruption. The introduction of electricity and artificial light has shifted this and now most artificial light serves to wake us up and inhibit sleep. This revolutionary invention prevents our bodies from producing melatonin to help us sleep at the right time.

Our world bombards us with blue light – light bulbs, TVs, computers, phones, clocks, radios and backlit devices. Evidence shows that *removing* blue light for at least 1 hour before sleep is the most effective way to create sufficient melatonin for sleep conditions. Simply reducing exposure to blue light is not effective because the smallest amount of blue light can suppress melatonin production in the brain.

Managing your exposure to blue light will help you fall asleep and achieve a state of deep sleep more quickly. It will also allow you to go back to sleep quickly when you are woken in the middle of the night.

You can still have your modern life and conveniences, while minimising your blue light exposure before sleep time. And for so many mums, whose lifeline is their smartphone and Facebook in the middle of the night, you can still continue to do that and manage your blue light exposure, if you do it properly.

The quickest and funniest way to eradicate blue light exposure is to get yourself a sexy pair of amber safety goggles. I am serious! I have two pairs – one for over my glasses and a nicer slimmer pair for when I choose to have my glasses off. (http://geni.us/NightShades) These are specially designed as workwear to protect the eyes from blue light emitted from welding arcs. Research from 2009 demonstrated significant improvement in sleep quality and mood from participants who wore amber safety goggles for 3 hours before bedtime over a 1-week period[138].

If you use a smartphone, enabling "night mode" will put an amber hue on the screen to reduce the blue light emitted massively. This can be set automatically to come on and turn off at specific times of the day. I

---

138 Burkhart K, Phelps JR. Amber lenses to block blue light and improve sleep: a randomized trial. Chronobiol Int. 2009 Dec;26(8):1602-12. doi: 10.3109/07420520903523719. PubMed PMID: 20030543.

suggest you have it on at least 7pm to 7am, this will allow you to use your phone during the night if you wish without waking you up even more.

Change the lightbulbs in the lights you use at night. For example, get a red or amber light for the hallway, bathroom and bedrooms. These will emit enough light for you to see without inhibiting your melatonin production, allowing your body to continue in sleep mode.

These tips also work really well for older children and improve the quality of sleep of other people in the house too.

12.3.2   NOISE

Night-time outside of the womb is a totally different place to that of the unborn baby. When in utero, your baby can hear all the sounds of your body. In relative terms, these sounds are as loud as putting your ear inches away from a running power lawn mower and louder than your vacuum cleaner. Dr Harvey Karp explains, "Parents intuitively use the right pitch to soothe their baby's cries. They start by making a loud, hissy shhhh sound and then gradually lower the pitch and volume as their little one relaxes into sleep."[139] In the same article, he writes that white noise is important for all babies as they learn to adjust to the world outside the womb and around them. White noise should start loud, when baby is crying so that they can hear it, and then become quieter and deeper in sound as they settle.

A practical way of implementing this to help your baby sleep is to *shhh* loudly and strongly at first, when they are awake, perhaps unsettled. As baby quietens and settles, you gradually soften the *shhh* and quieten it. You can employ this technique when baby stirs during the night too – before you pick them up, *shhh* loudly and noticeably, see if they respond, and then quieten again as they settle back to sleep. This will not work if baby is in pain.

12.3.3   DISTRACTIONS

---

139 https://www.happiestbaby.com/blogs/blog/baby-white-noise-mistakes

There is such temptation to get distracted when feeding baby and catch up on TV, emails, browse your phone, etc. Yet, doing all this takes away from baby and feeding.

If you are breastfeeding, you should *always* be aware of baby's latch, especially in the early days, and even more so if baby has had a tongue-tie release. There are multiple benefits in taking the time to focus on your baby when doing the bedtime feed (although this also applies to all other feeds).

Firstly, by constantly being attentive to baby's latch, there is a greater chance of baby swallowing less air, and as a result, having less air to pass through their little body and less discomfort later in the night.

If you are bottle-feeding baby, it is just as important to pay attention to the latch on the bottle teat. If you see baby spilling or dribbling, then the latch is not sufficient and baby is drinking air. If their latch is forming a proper seal around the bottle teat, air cannot get into the mouth to be swallowed with the milk. If there is dribbling or spilling, you know air will be getting in because milk coming out.

In this situation, I suggest trying a different range of bottle teats to find out which works best for your baby. There's unlikely to be one answer for every baby, so trial and error is the best way here. Constant initial effort will pay off, because the proper latch will become baby's natural latch soon enough, though you should always pay attention.

Secondly, by removing distractions from the feed, bedtime feeds become a place of sanctuary, safety and quiet. Phones, TV, tablets and other devices cause noise and distraction for your baby, not just for you. Let baby focus on the task in hand. And it's not good enough to plug in earphones, because the light from our devices disturbs sleep patterns. Remove them from the room for the bedtime feed.

Thirdly, mindful feeding will allow you to change baby's latch every time your little one slips off or back to their "old ways". It also allows you to take stock of your amazing baby. Let these feeding times be joyful and happy. So often with babies who are up all night, the rest of the time is so difficult, so hard, so exhausting and so stressful that we don't take time to just look at our little miracles. Try this at bedtime tonight:

For one feed, focus totally and completely on your baby.

Gaze on ***them*** and notice every inch of ***their*** face. Memorise ***their*** beauty. Congratulate yourself on your little miracle of life.

For one feed, forget the long day and do not think about the night ahead.

For one feed, focus on the present, a happy suckling baby.

For one feed, smile and enjoy everything about ***yourself*** and ***your baby***.

Connect, breathe and be thankful.

Baby has an ability to sense mood and energy. In the same way that you can walk in on an arguing couple, even when they're not voicing their argument at that moment, you can sense and feel that something is not right. Baby can do that too. That is why it is important for you to look after yourself and your energy. By protecting yourself, you protect your baby.

Wind frequently during the feed, more so if baby is having milk from a bottle. Try to get as much of the wind out as possible. Try not let baby fall asleep when feeding and make sure they have a full feed before going to sleep. Once the feed is finished, let them go to sleep. Pay close attention because baby may want to suckle whilst falling asleep which is not the same as feeding when falling asleep.

12.3.4   Where Baby Sleeps

When it comes to where you and baby are sleeping, make it easy for yourself. If your baby is in their own room and waking frequently, I strongly suggest that you change this. You should be sleeping as close to your baby as possible. You can achieve this in a number of ways, so choose the one that works best for you.

You can co-sleep. The normal rules apply to co-sleeping:

- Make sure your baby cannot:
  o   Fall out of the bed
  o   Get stuck between the mattress and the wall
- Make sure that bedding doesn't cover their head or face
- Keep the bed cool by using blankets rather than a duvet
- Put baby to sleep on their back
- Keep your pillow clear from baby's head or face
- Put yourself between your partner and your baby. (Mothers have an in-built instinct to not roll onto baby. Fathers do not.)
- Do not co-sleep if you have consumed any alcohol.

If you don't want to co-sleep, a bed-nest is another option, and one of the best options in my opinion and experience.

If you have the space, you don't even need a special bed for baby. Simply remove one side of their cot bed and push it right up beside yours. You do need to be wary of your duvet getting pushed over onto your baby.

The fabulous benefits of both co-sleeping and bed-nest arrangements are your feet don't have to touch the floor when tending to baby during night wakings. You don't even have to leave your bed. Psychologically, this was biggie for me. With the action of getting out of bed, walking to baby's cot or another room, you are waking your body up more and more, which means difficulty getting back to sleep when baby settles. I understand that there are sometimes points during the night when walking around the house is the only thing that will help and I have more on that later.

The additional benefit of a bed-nest arrangement is that you get peace of mind that you're not going to roll onto baby and can hear baby sleeping, so you'll know when they wake. You don't have to have additional monitors and technology in the bedroom, which also contribute to sleep disruption.

If baby is in a cot, have the head of the bed propped up by about 4 to 6 inches. **Do *not*** do this with a pillow, but get something solid that you can put under the feet at one end of the bed. Ensure it is sturdy and baby's mattress remains flat on their bed; I've used books and timber myself.

If you can fit their cot into your room, do so. The less distance you have to physically move to get to baby during the night, the easier it will be on you.

TIP: Unless baby has a dirty nappy, it does not need changing in the middle of the night. Buy the next size up (if it's not way too big) for night-time nappies and this will have the extra soakage room to keep baby's bottom dry throughout.

Now sleep soundly until baby wakes you, whether that's half an hour, or an hour and a half. Trust that your baby will wake you, they have done every night so far. And if you are worried, invest in a baby movement sleep sensor like Angelcare http://geni.us/AngelCareSleep.

12.3.5   GOING TO SLEEP

With young babies under 6 months, I believe there is nothing wrong with baby going to sleep on you. Baby is not manipulating you by wanting to be as close to you as possible. This is a natural bonding instinct that baby has been given.

You may find it hard, but look at it from baby's perspective. Before baby was born, all they knew was warm and cosy and protected. They knew mum. During birth, they went through the most traumatic event they've ever experienced. Regardless of how much they might want to, they cannot go back. Their eyes may not be able to focus yet, but the lights are brighter. Their ears may not yet have crystal clear hearing, but everything is louder than it was before. The protection baby once had is gone and they are exposed.

But baby knows *you*, Mum. You are their protector. You are the one constant in their life. Your voice was always there and it is still here now. Baby recognises your movements and knows it's you holding them, senses your smell more strongly and gets reassurance that it's you. All of these soothe them. Just being in your arms and close to you soothes your baby.

If baby is hungry, they know you will feed them. If they're tired, they know you will help them sleep. If they are hurting, they know you will do your best to fix it. And that on its own is enough. Baby knows that you are enough. *Trust* yourself that you are enough too. *Know* that you are enough.

So when it comes to sleeping, if baby wants to sleep on you, and you know they'll go to sleep on you quickly, don't fight it. Let your wee one fall asleep and then gently lay them down in their sleeping place.

This should be about 7-7:30pm. If you have been in a dark room, being mindful and quiet for the last 30 to 60 minutes with baby as they fed, then you are probably pretty sleepy too. What I'm going to write next is *really important*, so pay attention.

GO TO SLEEP.

Right now, more than any other time of the day or night, it is crucial that you go to sleep. Even if it's only for half an hour. By being in the sleep environment for the last hour, your body and mind are ready to rest. There is melatonin rushing around your brain and your mind is relaxed and poised for sleep. Forget about your husband's dinner! He can have a boiled egg if he wants. Lie down beside your baby and close your eyes. Your body will thank you for it. This might be your highest quality sleep of the night because you are so well prepared for it.

12.3.6   MANAGING NIGHT-TIME WAKING

There's no two ways to say this. Night wakings are a bitch. They drain the energy from the baby's sleep. If you're getting out of your bed to tend to your baby, they will be waking you up too.

These tips for managing wakings come from my personal experience, so they may be different for your reality:

1. Co-sleep or bed-nest. When baby stirs, you are beside them already and don't need to put your feet on the floor to resettle them. You get more time in your own bed, even if this means dad sleeps somewhere else for a little while. Sharing a bed with your partner is not always best if it means neither of you are going to be rested.

2. Try this: if you hear baby stirring and you believe they are not yet hungry and don't seem to be in pain, comfort them back to sleep with *shhh* and patting before they fully wake. This can teach them how to self-soothe between their sleep cycles. With older children, leave them a few minutes before tending to them to see if they will self-soothe back to sleep.

3. Leave your phone in a different room.

4. Change the lightbulb in your bedroom to a red or amber light to remove blue light.

5. Only change baby's nappy if necessary.

6. Keep a bed mat under where baby sleeps and a stash of fresh ones beside the bed to minimise time and disruptions during the night if you need to change the bed. If your baby is sleeping in their own bed, layer waterproof sheets and cotton sheets so that a bed change is simply removing one set each time.

7. Accept the normality and blessing of your baby waking during the night. Have confidence that your body will cope with disrupted sleep. It is evolutionary that babies wake during the night, so it's really a good sign (even if it does not feel like it right now). In fact, Dr James McKenna believes that frequent night wakings are protective from SIDS (Sudden Infant Death Syndrome), and life-threatening sleep apnoea[140].

8. If you suspect baby is in pain with trapped wind or other abdominal discomfort, immediately start tummy massage and

---

140 James J. McKenna; Night waking among breastfeeding mothers and infants: Conflict, congruence or both?, Evolution, Medicine, and Public Health, Volume 2014, Issue 1, 1 January 2014, Pages 40–47, https://doi.org/10.1093/emph/eou006

cycling of legs, do not wait it out for an hour and hope it goes away by itself.

13 RELATIONSHIPS AND REFLUX

An unsettled baby changes everything.

Whether from reflux, silent reflux, colic, food intolerances and allergies, illness or anything else, if your baby is totally unsettleable, your life changes more than you could possibly imagine, and in a way that makes it impossible for most other parents to relate to you. Reflux makes *everything* so much harder.

In this chapter, where I use the word "reflux", the cause doesn't matter. This chapter is about what having an unsettled baby means for your relationships.

When I first found out I was pregnant, I was so excited about being a mum. I was scared about the prospect of being 100% responsible for the life of another human being, especially with reflection on my own life to date! At times, I felt I'd truly struggled to look after myself, often neglecting my own health, forgetting to eat, not bothering to sleep, sometimes not even going home at night. (Shock horror!)

And in a few months, that was all going to have to change. Those seemingly little things in life wouldn't be tolerated by a baby who *needed* me. And while I was more than scared about my ability to step up to the mark, I was truly looking forward to it with every inch of my being. Deep down, I *knew* I had the ability to do this, *to be a mum.*

Yet still, I was not prepared for the *level* of change required, because my baby had silent reflux. My little Sunflower was only 16 hours old when I was first told to "quieten your baby". That was our first night together, and one of the loneliest and longest nights of my life. I was alone, without my husband, in a hospital, with my newborn baby girl. She had been born at 7:11am, and I'd been awake all day, so when 9pm came and her dad was sent home to get some rest, I was hoping for some too. But Sunflower did not rest. She didn't sleep except on my boob or in my arms.

Every time I moved her back to her cot, she screamed. Picking her up onto my shoulder, she settled again. Every 20 minutes, I thought she was asleep, would lie her back down, but within minutes she'd scream again.

I walked the corridors with her, I sang to her, I cried with her. I was asked by the midwives to move away from the ward where other new mums were trying to sleep so that she would not disturb them; that I needed to realise the other new mums were exhausted and needed their sleep. I was told to take a bottle of formula and give that to her.

I did not receive help.

I did not get any positive support.

I did not get any hugs.

I did not get anyone telling me that everything would be fine.

I did not have anyone ask if Sunflower was okay.

I did not have anyone spend time with us to see what might be going on.

I was caught napping in my bed with Sunflower in my arms and told she needed to sleep in her cot. Five minutes later, we were both up and about again. It must have been 5am when I finally gave up and fell asleep in my bed holding Sunflower. I know I didn't sleep deeply or well. And I was counting the minutes until 9am when J would come back and look after me. I may have texted him to be waiting outside the door to get to us as quickly as possible.

When he arrived, I must have fallen apart. He had slept, thankfully, but from that point on neither of us was going to sleep like we used to for years to come...

13.1   RELATIONSHIP WITH ME

My total lack of sleep meant that I was beyond reason, so far beyond the line of reason that it was a dot. I had zero control over my emotions, and zero awareness of that. I was a bitch to live with. I don't remember it like that; yet I know it's true.

I couldn't reconcile the immense love I felt for Sunflower and the overwhelming desire for her to be different. I didn't blame her for not sleeping, for wanting me all the time, but I did resent her for stealing *every hour* of my being from me.

I lost myself completely. I was not the mum I wanted to be, nor the mum I thought I was going to be.

Looking back, I have become so much more than the mum I thought I would be, the woman I saw in my visions of mothering. That journey has been one I never imagined. And being the mum I am today is amazing. I am not perfect and I am happy with that. I do my best every day. Some days that is utter crap compared to other days and that is okay too. Before being a mum, if I could have envisioned the mum I am today, I would surely have said, "Yes! I want to be her!" If I'd known the toil, anguish, pain and suffering to be here, I would have opted for being less of a mum but with an easier ride! Yet, it was not a choice. It was a strange kind of gift, but a gift nonetheless. And 5 years down the line, I can see that.

As I was going through it, though, I couldn't handle my own feelings of shame, guilt and not coping. I quashed them every day, rose above them every day. And doing so alone.

In the years since becoming a mum, I have grown in ways I never thought possible. I have *patience* for the first time in my life. In my previous professional career, I could often be heard saying "patience is a virtue I do not possess", but I can honestly say I'm incredibly patient these days. It was something I had to learn to remain sane. To put up with watching my baby in pain, every day and every night, not being able to do anything about it. To know that eventually sleep would come to us both. And to just know to wait it out. To keep holding and reassuring my crying baby. To not fall over.

Becoming a better mum through my baby's reflux has made me a better person. It has taken years. It has made me more vulnerable. It has opened my eyes to seeing the world in a different way. It has made me ask the stupid question time and again, until I am happy with the answer. It has made me refuse the status quo, because I know my child and I know what I see. It has brought greater observational powers to me. It has made me trust my eyes, my ears, my heart. It has brought me in touch with my gut instincts. I know what I see and I know what my baby is going through.

Reflux has made me want to help my child by moving mountains. I have moved mountains.

Reflux has battled with me to find so much more in reserve that at breaking point I stood up instead of falling over. If this had been my life, I would have accepted so much less. This was not about me. This was about my greater calling for the life and health of my baby. As custodian of her health and protector of her life, I was duty-bound to do better, ask better questions and find better solutions.

Reflux made me, after it tried to break me.

Be gentle with yourself. Trust yourself. Know that this is not your fault. You *will* get through it and be a stronger person for it.

13.2   PARTNERS & HUSBANDS

Reflux drives a stake through the heart of your relationship with your partner, be it marriage or other.

Before your baby arrived, you and your partner had time for each other. You probably realised that by having a baby you would have less time. You decided that was going to be okay because you were bringing another person into your family, together. And whether you spoke about it or not, you knew you would find your own way to make family life work. You were looking forward to it.

The first few days are amazing. You are in awe of what you've both accomplished. Family and friends visit from everywhere, and everyone wants to see you and your new baby. After these days are done, you sit down and realise just how exhausted you are. I remember resenting everyone getting time with my baby except me.

When people asked how she slept (only days old), I would say "she doesn't", and would get the same reply from everyone. "Sure that's normal. She'll settle down soon enough. Enjoy her while she's so little. They grow up so fast."

The days turned into weeks, and the weeks turned into months, and she did not settle. She did not sleep. She screamed a lot. And that time together that J and I longed for never came. Every night, he would come home from work. I knew the struggles, mental and emotional, of the corporate environment where he worked, but I was still so jealous that he got to speak with big people every day. Just as he longed for the time he could do baby-talk.

But our Sunflower didn't want her daddy. She wanted her mummy. All the time.

When J would take her to give me a break in the evenings, she would scream louder. Screaming in pain was one thing, but coupled with "I don't want to be in your arms; I want to be in her arms", that cry is heart-wrenching.

I can only imagine what it's like for a father not to be wanted by his own child.

So for J to have Sunflower time, which wasn't quality time at all, it was squats and lunges all the way to help her settle. To give me a little break, he had to carry my clothes, preferably dirty clothes, so that Sunflower could be fooled that mammy was closer than I really was.

The consistency of the crying and screaming, the surety that it was going to be all evening, every evening without fail, and the certainty that

my arms were the only place she'd sleep drove a baby wedge between us –
both physically and metaphorically.

Keeping my emotions bottled up made everything far worse. The strain
on our relationship was immense.

I know now, if I'd just trusted him, allowed my vulnerability to be
shown to just one person, he would have been my rock without fail.
Instead I built a massive fucking wall between us. One that has taken some
effort to tear down.

Reflux can put so much strain on a relationship that the relationship can
fail completely. I've seen it happen and it breaks my heart. And I can see
why it goes that way.

I treated my husband like shit. I didn't do it on purpose. I was not a
rational being. I can see that now, but if I'd been told this when I was in
the middle of it, I would probably have punched the messenger. Hard. In
the balls.

J understood. For that, I know I'm lucky. Some partners don't always
see or experience your reflux baby the way you do. Some partners see a
sleeping baby at night, because baby is so worn out from screaming in pain
and crying all day. Some partners work all day and simply don't have the
same frame of reference as you do.

This is why being totally **_honest_** and **_vulnerable_** with your partner is so
important. There are couples for whom reflux has ended their relationship
completely. It is serious. Communication with your partner is critical.

Be kind and gentle to your partner. Ask for help and _let them help_. Be
vulnerable. Allow yourself to feel supported.

13.3   RELATIONSHIP WITH BABY

You may feel torn in two completely opposite directions when it comes to your reflux baby and wonder how it's possible to love and hate so passionately at the same time.

You love your child, no doubt.

And you hate this reflux that is overshadowing your every minute.

You love your baby and you hate that you can't take away their pain.

You love your baby and you hate that they are a permanent attachment to you.

You love your baby and you hate that you can't even go to the toilet for 2 minutes without them screaming.

You love your baby and you hate the loneliness of being a reflux mum.

You love your baby and you hate the comments you get from unwitting strangers.

You love your baby and you hate your friends' babies' ability to sleep.

You love your baby and you hate everything else about being a mother.

An unsettled baby is one of the most challenging sorts of children. At least if they were ill, you would get help from a doctor. If they had a fever, you would be taken more seriously.

I despaired every day. I would go out for tea or juice every day. I would force myself to leave the house, just to leave the house. And it was so hard.

The one thing that kept me going was my baby. I did everything for her. I survived each day and night for her. I hated her reflux for not letting me sleep. Even though I did not know it was reflux.

I used to cling so tightly to her at night. I would hold her close and sing through the tears so that she would eventually fall asleep in my arms and then I would rest my eyes for 5 minutes until I needed to sing again. I never doubted my baby and I always trusted what I observed.

Now 4 years later, Sunflower and Daffodil know that no matter what is going on with them, they can trust me to look after them. They know that I cannot take pain away. They know they can get comfort from my hug.

For reasons of mere survival, I became an attached parent. In more ways that I ever imagined I could be attached. You may have heard of the Velcro Baby. This is both of my girls. And if nothing else, I can say 4 years later that my relationship with my kids is stronger than I ever believed it could have been.

I trust them. They trust me. Unconditionally.

I have learned that babies and children rarely *want* to misbehave. Sure, there are times when they are testing boundaries, but I can read these situations. I understand what is going on for them. In truth, I can honestly say that being a reflux mum has made me a better mum. A stronger mum, a patient mum, a fiercer mum, a trusting mum.

Now that they have outgrown the reflux, I have amazing relationships with them both. I sincerely mean it when I say that everything I did, even giving up my identity for them, has been worth it.

They have brought out the best in me, and indeed the worst at times, and I'm a better person for it.

13.4   RELATIONSHIP WITH EXTENDED FAMILY

Reflux makes a mockery of you and your family. Your siblings, parents and in-laws do not, cannot understand what it is like to be a day or a night in your shoes, in your bed. They have never had a reflux baby themselves. And when they were parents, the culture around parenting was totally different from what it is today.

From personal experience, getting other people to help is difficult. It felt like it was impossible.

My husband understood. But my mother did not, his mother did not, my sister did not, his brother did not. We were lucky with my brother-in-law; he and his wife were the only people who supported us in doing whatever we felt was best and right for us and our baby. They were the only ones we felt didn't judge us for how we responded to our baby's every cry and whimper. They were the only ones with whom we could talk about how we truly suffered every night. They were the only ones who believed us.

When it comes to dealing with other members of your family, especially those who are supposed to "help" you, I offer the following approach:

- People tend to not accept that babies are different now to how they were when the last generation was born. And the thing is babies aren't different, but the *knowledge* we have is.

- Remember that all parents do the best they can with the information they have at the time. Just because you are perhaps doing something differently doesn't make what they did wrong. This is often an internal assumption that is not voiced. Believe me, being more understanding to potential upsets in others is a quicker way to an easier relationship.

- Explain that your baby isn't able to properly digest <insert offending food> right now. Ask the person to please switch to foods baby can digest. Remind them that there will be a time when your baby can have <insert offending food>. Just not yet.

- You may need to draw the line. If the person is not respecting your wishes about what to feed your baby, you may need to ask them to take a step back from the help they are offering because it is not helping. In fact, it is causing more harm to your child.

The hardest part is trying to be the bigger person. It's so difficult to hear totally unhelpful advice. Believe that all the advice people offer comes from a place of good intention. Remember they have no experience of what you're going through. If they have had experience, you may well be lucky to have an understanding family member to support you.

What can you and your partner do with this? What can you do to help?

Individually or together, you can sit down with the offending family member and explain that your baby is not like "normal" babies, that your baby is in constant pain and that you understand how difficult it is for people who do have first-hand experience of reflux/CMPA/food intolerances to know what life is like.

Ask them to trust you in everything you do. Ask them to stop offering advice because you have tried it all already. Tell them that if they truly want to help you, they will trust you. They will ask you how they can help. And they will do exactly what you ask when you ask for help and on your terms.

Sometimes this might be a prescriptive way of preparing some food. It might be a non-descript "please take baby for a walk" with a strict instruction to pick baby up if they start to cry, because they are more comfortable on someone's shoulder. Explain why these things are important.

Explain that if they can help you on your terms, this will support the trust that is needed with your relationship for the next few years as you guard your baby with your life, as you learn how to prepare food that will not aggravate an allergy or intolerance.

Spell it out that if they do not do as you ask, you will end up avoiding them and not asking for help. And you know this because it's what has happened in so many reflux families before you.

I would love to tell you that this approach worked with my family. It did not because I did not have the knowledge or strength to have these conversations. Since then, I've come to believe that if I'd known to have these conversations, they likely would have helped.

As my kids have ongoing allergies and food intolerances, these sorts of conversations are still pertinent in our life. The result of infringements – like letting my child having a sausage for dinner in a café – leads to grandparents not minding my kids. Because the result is a few nights where my daughter has sleep apnoea and I must stay awake making sure she keeps breathing. All from a bite of sausage.

It is not worth risking your baby's health and happiness, or your own sanity just to "keep the peace" or be friends with everyone. This is not your job right now. Right now, your job is to prioritise the health and happiness of *your* baby, *your*self and *your* family. If others cannot support you, you are better off without their "help". This may seem harsh, but it's true.

You can explain to extended family members in a positive way how they can help you:

- Ask them to stop passing seemingly insignificant comments, because these are not helpful.
- Ask them to stop assuming you haven't tried all the tips and tricks that have ever existed. You **have** heard them before. So many times. Instead, ask that they trust you when you say you've really truly tried everything and that you will ask for help if you need it. And when you do, you are opening the conversation to check you have tried everything.
- If they do happen across information that might be new, ask them to position it as such, to phrase it in this way, specifically so that you have the right to say no and they should not be offended by that. *There is stuff you may not have come across yet.* They have a free pass to make a suggestion using this phrase once a month. Set it at that. Agree to that. Agree that once a month you will listen to their suggestions, because they might actually have something valuable to add.

Doing this can open up great pathways of communication – you are open to genuinely listening, and they may have already filtered out loads of crap for you so they have the real nuggets of gold. Set a time limit for conversations. Do not slam or even comment on anything they say. At the end, thank them for their suggestions, even if you think they are total rubbish. Especially in the case of grandparents – they *do* have the best interests of your child at heart; they just might not be aware of how their interactions are affecting you.

13.5   RELATIONSHIP WITH FRIENDS

Reflux makes enemies of your best friends. It's not intentional on anyone's part. An unsettled baby is isolating, when really what you need is support and trust. I will say it again – only people who have had a reflux baby know what it is like to have a reflux baby. And really, I extend this to unsettled babies for all reasons.

Your friends who do not have babies do not understand. They are still allowed to believe that all babies are cute and gorgeous (which, of course, they are).

Your friends who are thinking of babies are allowed to believe that all this cuteness and gorgeousness is what is waiting for them. They are allowed to think all babies sleep through the night. They cannot possibly be expected to know that you can actually tell the difference between a painful cry and a "normal" baby cry when you hear one. And that there is no way on this earth that you, as a parent, would never let your baby "just cry" when it's a painful cry. And that's okay. That is their view on life.

Your friends will not understand why you've suddenly gone from being a social, outgoing and engaging person to someone who never returns their text messages, especially when you post beautiful pictures of yourself and your baby in nice places. If you are on social media, think of the images and information you are posting. Are you posting the cute pictures of your amazing baba? Are you posting the tasty hot chocolate you have managed to squeeze in when baby finally fell asleep after a long walk? Or are you posting hour-long audio clips of your screaming child? Or doing live video of the 2-hour 2am bounce-and-walk, scream-to-settle sleep technique?

Be honest with yourself. Your friends will only see what you put out there. If you are not telling them how hard your life is, they only have the information you tell them to go on.

Maybe a few very close friends are in the know. And maybe they feel helpless because they can offer you nothing but an ear and a shoulder, and only at weekends or in the evenings when you are doing bedtime. And only for a couple of hours, as they are still working Monday to Friday.

So that leaves your antenatal group of friends, or friends you've met if you've braved any baby classes. But maybe not. Because maybe you went to a class or two and your baby hated it so much you felt embarrassed to go back the next week. And because maybe, even assuming you got on with those in your antenatal group, you had a first few weeks of people returning your emails at 3am or that WhatsApp chat you sent, but not so much anymore. You might be lucky and have a group of ladies who are supportive and understanding, even if they don't have an unsettled baby themselves. They trust what you say. They understand your baby's cries of pain. They may witness it. They may have had their lounge puked all over. They, at least, can hold your hand for a while.

The isolation really kicks in when your reflux baby still does not settle after 4 months and you're still waking 6 or more times a night to tend to them. You realise you feel lucky, and thankful, if someone else isn't sleeping through the night. You feel like the world is against you when friends move on and you don't. You get increasingly sleep-deprived as the days merge together and the only place you can find solace is in Facebook groups and online forums. And when your new virtual friends say nothing other than, "It's okay, Mamma", that still means so much, because deep down you realise you are not alone. There are many, *many*, **many** other families going through what you are going through.

The best friends you can have right now is a support group of people who have either ***been there*** or ***are there*** with you. If you can find a local reflux group, that might be all the support you need.

14 REFLUX THROUGH DAD'S EYES

I am thankful to my wonderful husband for sharing our experience from his point of view. The following words have been written by J.

To the partners out there, from a dad...

I'm not certain my insights will change your experience, though I hope they will help you understand what it's like. And perhaps you will find better ways of helping your partner and baby.

Writing this, I know there will be things Áine remembers happening very differently. I know that I can't remember exactly what happened, as my memory of the last 5 years is patchy. Even now, I seem to remember the better parts more than the rubbish days.

As a dad, I want to make sure that parents, and if possible, families, understand that it is not just about mother and baby. As a dad, we go through our own life changes when we have kids, in my case most of them without any forewarning.

Our role in the first few months of baby's life is a supporting one, literally. This is even more important when a baby has reflux, as support is what your partner needs, whether they realise it or not.

My main advice is stick with it. It will get better. Just don't set your expectations too high with what is and is not possible. You will, as I did, learn to let life happen for a while and simply hang on.

14.1   IN THE BEGINNING

In hindsight, to say I was unprepared for the life-changing event of becoming a father, is an understatement. I had done the requisite reading of what would happen during the birth to try to prepare myself. I had discussed and understood the birthing plan with Áine. I had driven from home to the hospital at different times of day, so that I would have an idea of how long it would take. I'd spoken to friends who had children. I'd even planned how to get back from the hospital when we brought baby home for the first time.

I hadn't really given much thought as to what would happen then. I was not prepared for the all-consuming nature of having a baby around. For a routine that was 24 hours a day, 7 days of the week, with no breaks. While I have no direct comparison, from talking to other parents, I believe that having a reflux baby makes these life events even more intense. And this is made even more challenging when baby is only happy with her own parents. There's no time off for mum and dad. Especially for mum. Áine has had very few hours off in the years since we've had our kids.

Our relationship as a couple changed from chatting virtually every day about our lives, to barely seeing each other from one end of the week to the next. Even though we lived in the same house. Our lives simply became about surviving; looking after baby, tiding the house, preparing food and trying to get some sleep whenever possible.

From day one, our little Sunflower needed constant care and reassurance. All the advice we were getting was that "she just needed to learn to sleep", or "she's a colicky baby". We listened to our hearts and ignored this advice, and spent a lot of time holding and carrying Sunflower because this was where she was happiest, though not happy. This resulted in me and Áine not spending much time together at all. In the first 2 years of being parents, we went out for dinner *once* on our own.

We got into a routine where the best time for us to talk was when I was either driving to or from work while Áine was nursing or feeding baby.

14.2   From Memory

In truth, the first 2 weeks, as I remember, were tired as hell. We were keenly aware of the new life in our lives and the responsibility that came with it. All seemed normal and baby was waking, feeding and sleeping.

Though exhausted, I'd guess we were 2 weeks in when we began to realise all was not as simple as it should be. Baby was awake *a lot*. When she was awake, she was really unsettled or crying. Going anywhere in a car was a real trial, as Sunflower was clearly unhappy about being strapped into a seat and the position it put her in. She would literally scream from being put into her car seat until being taken out.

I remember many nights being awake until 3am with Sunflower while letting Áine get some sleep, going to bed when baby needed a feed just after 3am, getting up for work at 6am, then not getting home in the evening until 7pm, sometimes later.

And doing it all again.

I can remember some days thinking that I would not be able stay awake all day let alone drive home. During this time, my health suffered. I put on weight, eating the wrong food and suffering from real sleep deprivation. My performance at work was noticeably reduced, which introduced additional angst, as I was now the only salary-earner in our household. We'd also bought a house in the previous 2 years, which had turned into a much larger project than we had anticipated. So just trying to keep pace with the small maintenance jobs that needed to be done was really hard work.

I remember having so little time to do these jobs that none of my tools would get tided away properly, meaning the next time they were needed I couldn't find them. That meant more stress in an already difficult situation.

I found it impossible to understand why there were no real answers from anyone we saw. Doctors, midwives, health visitors, even the internet did not provide any real knowledge that was linked to what we were experiencing. Or provide any views on what we could do about it.

I was limited by the time I could spend seeing the professionals with Áine and this led to frustration – that generally came from her direction. It couldn't possibly be that all the professionals had no way of making a difference. This is, of course, not quite true in that the advice we were given was our baby just needed to settle herself and learn to sleep.

In time, she would grow out of it, we were told.

Very frustrating when all I could see was a baby and wife in distress, all of us getting more and more exhausted. We were in a downward spiral of frustration and despair. Luckily, we ignored the advice, comforted and held our baby, and kept on looking for a solution.

This all changed in the wee hours of a Saturday morning when Áine happened to find a website describing silent reflux. From that moment, we changed everything we were doing.

She tried a few things and they made an instant difference. This gave her and us more confidence in a way to improve our baby's life and our sanity. This was a real turning point for us, and since then everything has steadily, slowly gotten better.

I will say here, there is no quick fix. It took us a lot of time and energy to figure out what was going on and what to do about it. We hope this book will help provide some of the real basic information that would have helped us find out what was going on with our baby sooner.

I have one memory in particular that captures how Áine was at times. We used wipes for everything to do with our kids. I can remember her giving me an absolute bollocking in front of my parents for not closing the packet of water wipes properly!

In that moment, I wanted to argue the injustice of the comment. Instead, I chose – and this was one of my better reactions – to completely ignore it. Áine will only be hearing about it for the first time when she reads what I've written in this book. For me, her reaction was unjustified and embarrassing because I was getting a telling-off in front of my parents. However, I'm glad I choose to ignore it, because the truth is she was not upset about the water wipes. She was upset because of the situation we were in. And on that day, all her frustration and upset was directed at me, over a subject that was completely irrelevant to what she was really feeling. I ended up doing this quite often in the first 2 years – not because it was the easy option, but because not reacting was the right thing to do.

When these situations arose, I always attempted to come back to Áine later to try to find out what was really going on.

14.2.1   WHAT CAN YOU DO?

I found it hard seeing Áine get more and more exhausted. Baby only wanted her mum. Mummy was the only one who provided food and comfort. When I tried to settle baby so Áine could get some sleep, she would cry for hours in my arms. I cannot even begin to explain how upsetting this was.

At times, it felt like I was being rejected by my own baby, made worse by not having any sort of relationship with my wife compared to before our baby was born. I felt powerless to give her a break, and powerless to settle and comfort my baby girl. In those hours – many at night on my own – I tried all sorts of things to settle her and a lot of time walking and gently attempting to rock our baby into contentment. None of which really worked. I can recall in the first 2 years only once when Sunflower fell asleep in my arms.

What I'm trying to say here is, as a dad and husband, I felt I was not doing a great job. Everyone was tired. We had no time for anything other than baby and food, and for me, work. As Áine became more and more tired, I honestly did not know how to help.

What I did do, though, was as much as possible: keeping the house tidy, which I did each day while Áine was trying to settle Sunflower and before I went to bed; washing and drying the clothes, preparing as much food as I could; managing the bills and finances; helping with the weekly food shopping; keeping the house and other things going while leaving her to focus on baby, and if at all possible, to rest.

In these times, I stopped going out and seeing friends. I did have to travel for work. As much as possible, I limited this to only one night a week. I found that leaving Áine for any amount of time only made her more exhausted. To my mind, it was the wrong thing to do; I was better spending my time supporting my wife and baby.

As a person, I became a bit lost. It was 4 years until I really starting to uncover who I am now, since before our kids arrived.

14.2.2   WHAT MORE COULD I HAVE DONE?

Hindsight often shows how obvious other decisions or actions are now that could have made a difference then. I am not sure what I could have done differently.

There were so few, if any, people that we met and talked to who had been through what we were going through. Those who hadn't had a baby with reflux offered lots of help! Only recently have I spoken to a few people who have experienced what we did and the parallels are staggering, such that their experiences are the same. It's frustrating because there is so little help available.

14.2.3   IF WE HAD ONLY KNOWN...

Until the day Áine found out about silent reflux, we did not even know it existed. I am sure that had we at least been aware there was something called silent reflux, we would have saved months of stress, worry and sleepless nights. Health professionals should take note of this – because from all of the interactions we had with them, silent reflux, or reflux, or CMPA were never mentioned.

If we had the knowledge that Áine has pulled together here, we would have been able to improve our baby's life much sooner. We would have been able to manage both her diet and Sunflower's symptoms, and identify what we needed to change in both people's food.

Each and every day I am constantly thankful and grateful that Áine has the strength of will and character to keep looking after our babies.

J

15 A LETTER TO PARTNERS

To the partners out there, from a mum...

Dear partner of an extremely exhausted mum,

I would love you to read this book. Dip in and out as you please, or go from start to finish. The information within it will help you understand what is going on for your baby, and help you and your partner connect.

I know a few couples who have ended their relationships because of the stress and strain introduced to their lives by reflux. I do not assume that you are those couples. The couples I knew who have ended their relationships were not those sorts of couples either. If you are close to the beginning of your parenting journey, please do not underestimate the potential strains reflux can bring. If you are a seasoned parent, I know you do not.

Our lives changed with our daughter, Sunflower. We knew that would happen. We did not know how much. Sunflower brought joy and new meaning to our lives, but also filled every night with dread, made me hate my husband at times, and made me believe that he had an easy life.

You see, my husband, J, got to go to work. He had the opportunity to leave the house. He did not have a new permanent attachment. Our Sunflower did not need him in the way she needed me. She didn't even care about him.

With 5 years of hindsight, I can see this was incredibly hard for him. I cannot imagine what it must be like to have your precious and magical baby completely reject you. I cannot imagine how hard it was to speak to me. I was beyond exhausted, tired from uncomfortable sleep before giving birth, and 36 hours awake with 8 hours of labour in the middle. (I know I got away lightly with this labour!) I was a night in hospital with no help and a baby awake all night leaving me shattered from the beginning.

J did everything he could. Yet in my eyes, he had the easier job. He got to speak to grown-ups. He didn't get puked on. He only witnessed the crying at night. He got hours off from it during the day.

Looking back, I know I could have made life a little easier for myself. I've written about that elsewhere in this book. Here, I would like to speak to how you can support your partner. And of course, it will be different for every parent, for every child. These are my tips.

1. Give her a hug and be supportive. Regardless of how emotional she is. Or isn't.

2. I hid my emotions deep. Really deep. Or at least I tried. By trying to hide these emotions, J couldn't talk to me, couldn't engage with me. I left him no route in. I have written about this earlier in the book: as mothers, we need to be vulnerable, open and honest with our partners.

3. Recognise your partner's challenges and never tell her she has the easy part. There is nothing easy about listening to your baby scream for hours at a time and being helpless to do anything.

4. Listen without judgement to her when she talks about her day and her complaints. When she says it's all okay, really check. Often it is not. Recognise that amidst the lack of sleep and feeding baby, yes, she is going out every day, or going to every class she can find, or cafes or walks, because she needs to find connection. She needs to know that she is not alone. You can help by finding a local mums group with reflux and colic experience. Help her find somewhere to go where she will be listened to.

5. When she says the doctor is an arsehole, believe her and support her. Acknowledge that regardless of experience, the mother of your

child is the expert in your child.

6. I am not saying that you should placate her. I am not saying that you should put her on a pedestal and do everything single thing she asks. But when it comes to managing your reflux baby, do not give up at the first, second or hundredth time of not being wanted by your baby. Especially from the age of 9 months. If mum is the primary carer, understand the ways she has found to do things to alleviate your baby's upset. And do things the same way. Not because your partner wants you to do it the same way, but because it is beneficial for your baby to learn the routine. Routine calms babies. Being able to predict what is coming next helps baby understand the world around them.

7. Reassure your partner that this is not her fault. Reflux is not anybody's fault. It happens. Support her in finding the best solution for your baby. Happier baby = happier family.

This is all purely about how you can support your partner in the easiest way throughout her journey. While yes, this is your journey too, this advice is to make it easier for you to support her immediately.

When you get some time, read this book too. You will learn what your child might be going through and be able to support your partner. Support is the greatest gift you can give her right now.

If your baby doesn't sleep a lot, if your partner is breastfeeding, if you're finding that you have an overly reactive and highly emotional partner, and you don't know what you're going to be greeted by when you arrive home, don't worry.

This is normal.

Remember, she hasn't slept properly in the length of time your baby has been with you, plus a few months of pregnancy. She is so far past the line of sleep deprivation that the line is a dot. And sleep deprivation is a known form of torture.

You may not be able to understand why, when you tell her to get a few minutes rest when baby is sleeping, she refuses to put her head down and instead does the dishes.

Remember, this is part of her. There is a subconscious part of her brain telling her that her home must be clean and tidy for her child. This is the nesting instinct that may have started before she even went into labour.

I experienced a **drive** to maintain a clean and tidy home, to get the chores done, to have food on the table and laundry cleaned. I felt an overwhelming urge to look after my husband and keep him happy and have him see that I was coping. I knew the logical and sensible thing to was to sleep, but I couldn't make myself.

Then I figured it out... If my house was sorted and clean and tidy and I had nothing else to do, then I would probably have slept. If I had had enough food in the freezer, and a food menu plan, then my husband wouldn't have felt so helpless, wouldn't have nagged me to get some sleep, would have been able to support even more.

I believed that the only time I needed help was the time I dreaded when no-one else could help me: my night-times, the breastfeeding through the middle of the night, the lack of sleep and the dealing with colicky crying, painful gas; the time I was up at night singing and dancing and bouncing to settle my baby girl.

In truth, if I had recognised at the time that **any help** during the day would have allowed me to rest, relax and sleep, if I had accepted that my job was a night shift one with interspersed day-time requirements too, then I may have been able to accept that help and look for it more readily. I had the start of postnatal depression that wasn't picked up, because at my 6-week check I was fine; I was like most other mums of 6-week-olds, and my health visitors assumed there was nothing wrong.

I'm not sure what the most important message is here. Perhaps I'm saying be easy on your partner and yourself. Speak to each other, hold your tempers. You are both stressed by being unable to comfort your baby. You are both exhausted from lack of sleep (and sex). You both may be a little jealous of the other's "job".

Most of all talk, talk, talk and then talk some more.

With love and kindness,

Áine x

PART 5

YOU ARE NOT ALONE

16 REAL STORIES FROM REAL MUMS

You are not alone. Sometimes reflux feels so lonely, so enduring that you may worry that life will never be better. Whatever is going on for you, however your baby experiences reflux, no matter what other people say, your journey is real.

Here, I will show you that there are other families, mums and babies going through tortuous times as well. Some amazing mums have agreed to let me share their stories so that you know you are not alone. I thank them all from the bottom of my heart for letting me publish these.

NOTE: Some names have been changed to protect identity where requested. The words remain true to real-life events, experiences and feelings. Where names have been changed they are indicated by *.

16.1   JESSICA & BABY

My baby boy, who was around 3 weeks old, kept throwing up his formula and my breastmilk, and we all thought it was acid reflux. Even his doctor said it was. We tried 3 or 4 different formulas and different medicines, but nothing was working. His throwing up got worst after about a week, when finally one night he threw up and my mother instincts told me it was not normal and to take him to the hospital ASAP.

I picked him up and ran to my husband crying my eyes out and told him we needed to go to the hospital. Well, we took him in and they did blood work and an x-ray and didn't find anything. I told them all the symptoms he was having and they said it sounded a lot like pyloric stenosis, but acid reflux has almost the same symptoms.

They couldn't do an ultrasound on him there, so we went to a children's hospital out of town where they did one. Sure enough, he had pyloric stenosis. He was admitted that night and had his surgery the next morning.

He had lost over 5oz, was almost back to his birth weight and was dehydrated to the point where they had to put the IV in his head. At 1 month old, he was 6lb 11oz, when he'd been 6lb 7oz at birth.

If your baby is around 2 or 3 weeks old and up a lot, and if it looks like it's the whole bottle, please don't wait. Take them in for an ultrasound. It won't hurt to get it to be on the safe side. My son recovered so well from his surgery that he's now 5 weeks old and 7lb 2oz!

He is eating well, holding down his food and having many dirty diapers! He hadn't had a dirty diaper in almost 2 weeks and I thought he was just constipated.

His doctor told me babies this young don't get pyloric stenosis and diagnosed him with acid reflux. I'm happy I didn't listen to her and brought him to the hospital. She pissed me off for misdiagnosing him, so I switched his doctor.

My son went through so much those few days and all I did was cry. He's doing 100% better now and even smiled at me today for the first time when I was playing with him.

16.2   LUCIE & JOSEPH

It took a year for us to fall pregnant; a year of heartache and longing to see those two lines on a pregnancy test, but in January 2015, there they were. We were going to be parents. I thought we'd done the hard part in making a baby, me hiding it from work for 5 months as I feared I wouldn't get the job I'd worked so hard for, plus getting through the pregnancy and the labour, but nothing could have prepared us for what was to come.

It sounds so dramatic, like we thought we were the first people to find having a newborn hard, but my God, it was a shock. Joseph was born with tongue-tie, and it feels completely alien to me when people talk about the first two weeks where "all they do is sleep". All he did was scream. I swear he slept maybe 6 hours in a 24-hour period. It was hell and we wondered what we'd done to deserve this.

Once we'd had his tongue-tie cut, I remember one week of feeling like it was coming together. Breastfeeding was going well and I felt okay. I remember the exact night it changed, the night silent reflux reared its ugly head in our third week.

My husband had been away with work for the day and I literally thought I'd conquered the world surviving a day alone at home with Joseph. That night he screamed every time we laid him down; he screamed after feeding, he screamed for hours and hours every evening after that. We tried everything. I must have gone to the doctor every few days begging for help. I was an emotional wreck, but I would not accept that my baby simply had colic and ride it out. My mum and I even took him to A&E one night as he'd screamed solidly for 5 hours, as if in agony.

Finally, a paediatrician agreed with my pleas that he had all the signs of silent reflux and we were prescribed medication. He was better for a while, but the screaming continued and after many more appointments at the doctors' surgery, we were prescribed a dairy-free milk, which seemed to help. I gave up breastfeeding, as the screaming and thrashing at every feed had given me such bad anxiety that I wasn't producing enough milk for him anyway. I was reduced to tears when he tried to feed, but clearly he wasn't getting what he needed.

Having survived tongue-tie, colic, silent reflux and CMPI, I myself was diagnosed with postnatal depression. By that point, I had started to recover though, having fought the diagnosis for so long. I didn't need medication by then.

Our little boy is 13 months now. I feel like I could write a whole book on how hard we found that first year, but I fear it wouldn't be a happy read and I'd much prefer to look back on that time as a chapter that's in the past.

So many people will say "don't wish the time away", but honestly, I wouldn't want to go through that time again for anything. Despite us not wanting Joseph to be an only child, we don't know how we'd do it all again. The thing we find most upsetting is how we had to witness each other pushed to the brink, taking it in turns to be the strong one, and just not knowing what to say or do to help each other in the darkest of times.

We're so unbelievably lucky to have a gorgeous, cheeky and fun-loving little boy, with a smile and character that has made him infamous amongst friends and family as our "Strong-willed Eyebrows". We wouldn't change him for the world, but if we could live those first few months again without the misery of tongue-tie, colic, silent reflux, CMPI and PND; we'd do it in a heartbeat, and we don't feel any guilt about that.

16.3   REBECCA & TOM

As a 37-year-old "career girl" as my nana described me, the anticipation of becoming a mum for the first time was both joyous (I didn't think I would be lucky enough to have children) and terrifying (enough of my friends and family had kids by then for me to have an inkling of the reality!)

Despite best laid plans of giving birth to the Café del Mar chillout classics in a birthing pool while being fed Jelly Babies, using the skills my hypnobirthing teacher had taught me, my baby was delivered by emergency C-section.

Born not breathing and whisked straight to resuscitation, it certainly wasn't the birth I'd hoped for, but after the initial drama he recovered quickly and latched on as soon as he was laid on my breast. The frightening start to motherhood was forgotten the moment I felt his weight and the touch of his skin on mine. He curled those tiny fingers around my thumb and I felt utterly complete, exhausted but complete. This was my purpose in life!

We were kept in hospital for a couple of nights due to the complicated labour, delivery and C-section. I remember Tom crying a lot. The nurses were great and took him for a couple of hours at night so I could rest. Everything was a bit of a blur; I was still suffering the effects of a 32-hour labour without sleep and the subsequent anaesthetic. The elation was more than enough to get through those first few days and I presumed the crying was just a newborn thing. After all, he'd had quite a dramatic entry into the world!

I was incredibly lucky that my partner had managed to arrange an extended period of parental leave coupled with working from home. I had also made some fantastic friends through NCT, all of whom lived in walking distance, which was fortunate given I couldn't drive for 6 weeks. Had it not been for this great support network, I'm not sure I would have had the strength to follow my instincts as the challenges over the following weeks unfolded.

The first week at home was a bit of a slog. I had an infection in my C-section wound, was taking pain relief which left me horribly constipated, and found myself unable to sleep. I cried, the baby cried, and he cried, and he cried. As the first week melted into the second, my partner and I tried every trick in the book to stop the crying, with rocking, patting, jigging, music, light, no light.

There wasn't a parenting manual or blog we didn't read in the hope of finding a solution. It wasn't so much the crying that upset me, it was the fact I could see that my baby was in pain. His little face scrunched up, fists clenched, knees drawn up to his chest. Arching his back and kicking when he was put down. At one stage, I even remember leaning over his crib with my boob in his mouth in the hope that he'd fall asleep!

At this early stage, we were having frequent visits from midwives and I was having regular checks with the doctor. At every opportunity, I talked about the crying and how I was concerned my baby was in pain. As Tom was a *very* healthy 10lb at birth (hence the C-section!) and he was feeding well and putting on weight, the crying didn't seem to concern them.

Responses I had ranged from "some babies just cry a lot" to "you career mums, you're so used to everyone doing what you want, having a baby just isn't like that!" Looking back now, I can't believe I accepted such lame reasoning. But I was a new mum, I was exhausted and these were experts; surely they'd know if there was something wrong?

I began questioning my own expectations about what motherhood was about. I remember my partner and I looking at each other one night having played "pass the screaming baby" for one too many hours, with a look of utter defeat on our faces. *What have we done? We had such a great life. Can we even do this?* I can't believe I felt that way about motherhood so early on in my child's life, but I felt so very helpless and tired. We both did.

It was the wise words of a new mum friend that I'd made that helped me to realise my instincts as a parent counted more than anything. I'd donned some lippy, put on a clean pair of jeans, and dragged myself to a play and stay session at the local children's centre.

Tom was having one of his particularly bad days and I nearly turned around and went home for fear of disturbing the peace, but my straight-talking Antipodean friend collared me and took me to her house, where she and her sister passed a still-screaming Tom back and forth, and persuaded me to go back to the doctor.

It turned out that straight-talking-Antipodean-friend's sister had experienced a similar problem with her first child. She too had had to jump through hoops to get anyone to take it more seriously than "first time mum anxiety". She told me I knew my baby and they didn't. I had to stick to my guns. I saw my GP later that day and he suggested it might be colic or silent reflux and prescribed infant Gaviscon. My sense of relief as I left the surgery was huge; finally someone was listening. Little did I know it was only the beginning.

The Gaviscon could only be administered in milk which meant I needed to express. Tom had been exclusively breastfed, but I found expressing difficult. Tom hated the bottle, and I had to persevere, but after a few days it was clear that the Gaviscon was not working. Tom was screaming even louder, not only was he still in pain, he was being made to drink out of a bottle. He was deeply unhappy and letting us know about it!

I was so low. I felt completely defeated. I called the health visitor to get her advice as to what to do next. She told me that I must have not read the label properly and that I must be doing it wrong! I put the phone down and I cried and cried and cried. I then had a shower, packed a bag for the day, put Tom in his pram and took the bus to A&E.

We lived in south-west London at the time and there was a special children's A&E there. I went to the front desk, screaming baby giving an active demo as to my obvious distress. I explained that my baby wouldn't stop crying. I was worried my baby was in pain and no-one would help me.

To be fair to the receptionist, she made little comment at what I am sure sounded like first-time anxious mum despair and I was sent to the waiting room.

I sat there for quite some time, Tom still screaming, me looking weary, everyone else making cheery comments like "he's got a healthy pair of lungs hasn't he!" while looking for an excuse to move to the furthest row of seats from the din as possible!

The triage nurse examined Tom and listened to how we'd ended up there, both in tears and at the end of our tether. She called the paediatrician who put us in a cubicle and said she wanted to observe for a couple of hours. She examined Tom and then watched Tom feeding, crying, feeding, crying, as she popped in and out. She agreed he was clearly agitated but seemed reluctant to believe that he always cried quite as consistently as she'd observed. Eventually, she prescribed Tom two medicines which could be given alongside breastfeeding; ironically, one sounded like an expensive brand of champagne (and by then I felt like a stiff drink was my only sanctuary!)

I returned home clutching the prescriptions, hoping they would help Tom and save my sanity! A few hours after the first dose, Tom was calmer. He didn't cry for long after being fed and I was afraid to believe their might be hope! Tom was cluster feeding at the time, and as his distress was always more pronounced after feeding, so it was immediately noticeable that there was a change.

With each dose and each feed, I could feel my baby physically relax. His body almost unfolded and softened, his face gradually smoothed from red, angry and furious to pink, contented and inquisitive. Within 24 hours, I had a different child. Within a few days we had the beginnings of a routine. I cannot tell you the relief.

As a couple, my husband and I were able to leave Tom with a sitter and go out for a couple of hours alone. We could enjoy our evenings together as a family. I was able to get more than 4 hours' sleep throughout the night – sometimes unbroken! We both started to enjoy being parents. More importantly still, it seemed to us that our little boy, for the first time, enjoyed being in this world.

Tom continued taking medicine for silent reflux until he began weaning properly, at which time the doctor advised me to begin reducing the doses, which I did with no ill-effects. We were obviously relived that his body no longer needed medicine to help it work properly.

No parent wants to medicate their child at such a young and vulnerable age, but when it comes to making the decision about your child being in pain or not, there is simply no decision to make.

Looking back on that horribly stressful time there are two things that stand out.

Firstly, the struggle to get the health professionals who were caring for us to take our concerns seriously. It seemed that as long as baby was "thriving" and vital signs were all fine, anything else which couldn't be measured was simply "new parent angst"!

Secondly, once we did have a diagnosis, it seemed that no-one felt that it was a condition that warranted much attention. The fact my baby was in pain seemed of little consequence!

My hope for other parents facing similar challenges in the future is that healthcare professionals will be more empathetic towards parents with babies who cry excessively, that they will investigate whether there is an underlying problem, and if there is, will treat it quickly, with compassion and with understanding. No parent should be made to feel that their concerns over their child's health are unimportant.

16.4   ANNA & LUCIEN

Lucien was born at 37+1 by C-section. I noticed quite quickly that he brought up a lot of milk when lying down after a feed, but initially I put that down to an underdeveloped oesophagus. Once he got into feeding (he was bottle-fed), we noticed that he vomited a lot, sometimes projectile vomiting, and became progressively more uncomfortable during feeding.

By about 4 or 5 weeks old, he would scream incessantly much of the time. During feeding, he would take a few mouthfuls, pull off, scream and writhe around, drink more, pull off, scream, and so on. At night from around 2am or so, he would wriggle, grunt and cry for hours in discomfort.

I knew Lucien had reflux as a friend's baby had had it for 2 years and we'd spoken about it a lot. We put him on thickened reflux milk, which did help, though the night-time discomfort and screaming when feeding continued. He was gaining weight well though – "thriving".

However, there were so many other reflux symptoms that I noted: persistent cough, frequent hiccoughing, problems feeding, back-arching, stuffing his fists in his mouth, pulling at his ears. I could hear him swallowing frantically sometimes, and then cry, as he brought up liquid and swallowed it back down again.

At around 8 weeks, we visited my GP who quizzed me about his symptoms – I had gone prepared with a full list, and a video of him feeding and screaming. As he was already on thickened milk, she prescribed ranitidine (rather than Gaviscon), but a low dose for bed-time only.

We didn't suspect an intolerance to dairy as he didn't have any other symptoms. The medication helped a bit, but when he was about 12 weeks old, he was back to screaming during day-time feeds and barely drinking.

After a few days, in desperation, I put him in the sling, gave him an extra dose of ranitidine and fed him upright. It worked perfectly and he fell asleep happy.

Back to the doctor where we talked about maximum dosing. I had already worked out what he could be on from the NICE guidelines online, but I wanted my GP on board. We carried on with the ranitidine, tracking his weight and increasing where necessary for a few months – and it worked brilliantly. I even managed to get him sleeping well with a little gentle help to resettle without feeds.

I was so complacent when we started weaning! When reflux is well-controlled, it's like it doesn't exist. You forget about it – or at least I did.

So we started weaning... I followed the principle that baby just has a bit of what you're having, modified where necessary. He wasn't that interested in being spoon-fed but loved tasty food he could handle himself. I had heard that certain foods weren't great for reflux babies, but I didn't give it too much thought as he wasn't noticeably reacting to foods after eating.

However, this coincided with what I thought at the time was a late sleep regression. He started waking at night, sometimes every hour, and instead of resettling gently as he had, he started to fight me – screaming, arching, pushing at me. He was often inconsolable.

He was heavy too by that point! Trying to rock a 9kg baby back to sleep was difficult. I didn't link his reflux flaring up to what he was eating for some time. He was probably almost 9 months old.

Cue total panic – I had no idea what to feed him. I could only work on trial and error. Often when things were bad, we would go back to just milk for a while. We had to do this many times over. We discovered certain foods that were safe and he liked them.

By this point, we had discovered Aine and I had trawled her every post on the reflux Facebook groups I was a member of to get hints for what to feed him. We had an initial chat on the phone and she gave me some clues as to what was going on, which I researched thoroughly.

Even so, we could never get things back to perfect even with safe foods and milk. He was miserable in the day-time, frequent bouts of screaming. He would settle and wake from every nap crying. Eventually, he got a cold which turned into a cough at night, which didn't go away for ages.

To the doctor again and I practically begged her to give us omeprazole. She was reluctant but I had been thorough with my research and list of symptoms. I told her it was affecting my mental health. And it was.

The transition onto omeprazole was painful – his symptoms were increasingly awful for about 13 days, then suddenly great. He was happy. He slept better, instantly. Such a relief.

Once things were calmer generally, it gave me the space to see when food triggered a reaction. Cheese noticeably – streaming nose, face rash. We thought he had a cold, but it came and went over a few days. With this in mind, I went back to the doctor and asked for a prescription dairy-free formula, which they prescribed along with a referral for allergy testing. There were still many foods that he found uncomfortable – and this was at 11 months of age – but we transitioned to the new formula over a period of a couple of weeks. After a while with a safe diet (and Aine's help), omeprazole and Aptamil Pepti 2 formula, we reached what I would say was a good place again.

Lucien is now 1 year old, has started nursery (another dietary minefield) and is doing well – but still on the medication and prescription formula.

Eventually, I'll summon the courage to attempt weaning off them. Of course, the allergy testing came back negative. He isn't technically allergic to anything, though still reacts to foods here and there. I'm hopeful we'll be able to get to "normal" over time…

16.5   LEANNE, MALACHY & LORCAN

I have three babies, two are diagnosed reflux and tongue-tie babies. I say diagnosed because my eldest child was not diagnosed for his tongue-tie, which caused us to end our breastfeeding journey prematurely at 8 weeks. I have never known pain like it. My poor nipples were destroyed.

Anyway, my second baby came along I had heard of reflux but didn't really know much about it. I thought reflux parents were few and far between, and quite honestly, I thought they were exaggerating how bad things were. I realised pretty quickly how very wrong I was, and my respect for reflux parents shot through the roof. I wouldn't wish it on anybody; seeing your baby scream inconsolably in pain while you helplessly, uselessly, try to comfort them is soul-destroying.

My second, Malachy, was my first reflux baby and he was left undiagnosed for over 5 months. I asked every midwife, health visitor, lactation consultant and GP that I could about why my baby screamed 24/7, why he breastfed every 2 hours, day and night, why he would never sleep for more than 20 minutes at a time and only when it was on someone's chest.

I got the same rubbish back: it's colic; he'll grow out of it; breastfed babies feed more often than bottle-fed babies; posseting is normal (which it is, but not to the extent we were experiencing); you're tired because you have two close together. All that mumbo jumbo. I felt like the world's worst mum. I couldn't enjoy this wonderful new person in my life because he just screamed at me. All. The. Time.

It took until 5 months to realise that he probably had reflux. Around the same time I realised he probably also had tongue-tie. He fed poorly. It was agony with every feed. My nipples never healed and we both absolutely hated feeding times. But he wouldn't take a bottle. We tried every bottle and teat we could find, and he refused them all outright, so an exclusively booby baby he was.

I think that's when my PND started, from around 3 to 4 months old, when it became clear a bottle wasn't happening; knowing that I was the only one that could feed him and knowing that every 2 hours I had to go through that agony all over again was difficult to accept in my head. It was mothering instinct versus pain instinct; mothering always won and suppressing that pain instinct to push through the feed was mind-bending.

Still, at the point of realising he probably had reflux, I didn't quite yet realise he had the tongue-tie, so I took him to the GP again and informed them that he had reflux. The GP looked incredibly taken aback at being so abruptly informed, but he actually asked me questions this time, unlike the others who just fobbed me off.

He agreed that it was indeed reflux, and the volume of sick alone was a concerning indicator, so he gave me Gaviscon to try for 3 to 4 weeks. It did naff all. I know it works for some babies, but it didn't work for us at all. Malachy ended up with a complete syringe aversion because I was constantly forcing one into his poor little mouth.

About two weeks after being diagnosed with reflux, I then realised he had tongue-tie because I saw it. I went to baby clinic in a flurry of tears and demanded they check him for tongue-tie, preparing myself for a battle. An exclamation of "oh yes, he does have a slight posterior tongue-tie" was quickly followed up with "but posterior is never as serious as anterior, and it's not affecting his feeding or weight gain, so we'll refer you to the local tongue-tie clinic".

They had completely failed to notice that he had dropped 2 centiles in 5 months, and ignored me when I said his feeding was poor. At the local clinic, we were informed that he was now too old to have the division through the NHS; my only choice was to go private or suck it up. Private was completely off the cards. We had no possible way of affording the £150 treatment at the time, so my only option was to suck it up, and continue to feed my baby on broken, cracked, bleeding nipples until he chose to wean off me. That was really hard.

Shortly after that, it was clear that the Gaviscon wasn't working, and we needed something else. Back to the GP we went, making sure we saw the same nice one who listened, and again he heard me and prescribed ranitidine. What he failed to mention, which was really quite important, was that the ranitidine had to be given 30 to 60 minutes before a feed. So, I gave it to him like I did Gaviscon, immediately before a feed, and of course it did nothing at all. And we still had the syringe aversion that was by this point getting worse – I have never heard a noise like that come out of a baby before or since, and it's not something I want to repeat.

By this point, I'd become completely numb to his screams. I heard them and responded like a robot. I didn't empathise with him at all. PND had well and truly taken hold.

After just two weeks of ranitidine, I went back to the GP and completely broke down. I ugly cried. Between sobs, I told him that nothing was working, could we please try something else and have a referral to a specialist because my child was broken, and I needed help to take his pain away and make him happy.

The GP reluctantly prescribed omeprazole and sent off the referral, and finally Malachy calmed down. The sick continued but the screaming didn't. We continued with it right up until the referral, at which point he was 10 months and should have been weaning off it.

Not realising this, the GP had put him on the highest dose possible, and continued to increase it with his weight. One side effect of the omeprazole that we didn't know about was insomnia. So instead of screaming in pain, he screamed from exhaustion.

He was also feeding every 2 hours, because his tongue-tie prevented him from eating successfully so he was always hungry. The GORD consultant was fantastic, not only did he give us advice about how to wean him off the omeprazole, but he also advised us on how to wean him off the breast and eat proper food. He came off the breast fairly well, but it took a further 8 months to get him to eat properly.

At 2 years old, he still has issues with many, many foods, something I firmly believe is because his mind associates them with the pain of reflux, of too-early weaning when he wasn't ready (on health visitor advice), and syringes being forced into his mouth.

On top of this, we were told he would be able to have his tongue-tie cut at 12 months under general anaesthetic. We were not offered an operation date until two months before his second birthday.

My reflux and tongue-tie experience with Malachy was traumatic. It left me with PND and almost no maternal bond with my baby. The entire process was isolating. At no point did I feel supported by immediate care professionals until I found that one GP who listened, but unfortunately listened too late.

Malachy didn't get omeprazole until he was 7 months old, by which point the damage was done. I have since gone through intense psychotherapy for PND and trauma, and I don't think I will ever be "over" it.

I cannot think of it without wanting to sob uncontrollably because I feel like I let down my baby, like I didn't fight hard enough for him, and angry with myself that I lost my way as a mother. In reality, I was a tired second-time mum with a 14-month-old and a newborn, and the professionals I turned to for help consistently let down my son. I have to remind myself regularly that that is not my fault.

When we became pregnant with our third, Lorcan, we said that we would never allow this to happen again. At the slightest whiff of reflux or tongue-tie, we'd be off to a new clinic to get diagnosed and sorted, and we put money aside for a private tongue-tie division just in case.

Lo and behold, he was a tongue-tie and reflux baby, so I did the GP and the breastfeeding clinic in the same week. Again, I was told that a posterior tongue-tie is not serious, particularly as he could stick his tongue out a little bit, and it wasn't duly affecting his feeding. (It was, he struggled to latch, and snacked constantly). As I was concerned and had experienced it before, they referred us.

The date of our appointment came the following week, and was set for two weeks away, making it three weeks from diagnosis. I was horrified and furious. They had seen my cracked and bleeding nipples, seen how he struggled to latch and feed. I'd told them that the only way we were getting sleep was to take it in 2-hourly shifts to sit up with him on our chests, making sure we stayed awake on our shifts by watching TV. How could they expect us to continue like this for another fortnight?!

I booked in with a private tongue-tie specialist, and got it cut 3 days later. On the scoring system, and from her own examination, she said he had one of the worst posterior ties she had come across, and sticking it out was no indication that it was not a serious tie. He was so tied that he was completely unable to lift his tongue, and therefore was completely unable to latch in any way effectively. I cried floods of tears from sheer relief.

My instinct had been completely right. His tie was severe! His tongue was snipped, he healed well and fed so much better. He was 3 weeks old at the time of his division.

Next was the reflux, this time it was silent. I had had the foresight to join some social media groups early on, so twigged it was silent quite quickly. I noticed a lot of parents say that silent reflux was harder to get a diagnosis for, so I went to my GP prepared for a fight. The GP attempted to dismiss my experiences, but I refused to back down. We were prescribed ranitidine after she consulted with a paediatric registrar at the local hospital, who stated that "reflux is over-diagnosed, he is probably just colicky, and reflux medication doesn't work anyway". I was utterly speechless and in fairness so was the GP. We set a time limit of 2 weeks for the ranitidine, and if it didn't work, then we'd try something else.

This time I administered correctly, but it was challenging as there was no routine to the feeds and very often we didn't make it to the 30 minutes which rendered that dose useless. It made no change to his pain, so we went back. This time I asked for lansoprazole, in an attempt to avoid the insomnia fiasco that was omeprazole.

Within a week of lansoprazole, I had a different baby. He did have some issues with constipation when we first moved onto it, but once his tummy got used to it, he would smile, feed and, more importantly, sleep.

What I found most frustrating during the process with both of my children was lack of diagnosis, lack of information, and wrong information. We were so utterly let down the first time around. We were given completely incorrect information both times. It was extremely confusing and utterly exhausting at a time where we were already cripplingly tired.

My constant thought with both babies was that it shouldn't be this hard to get treatment to prevent a baby's pain. As adults we can get it at the drop of a hat, and can understand and comprehend our pain. Why can't we give that same level of care to these tiny little people? It utterly broke me that Malachy spent the first 7 months of his life in horrendous pain every single day.

I think the most important thing for parents to take away from my story is to listen to your instinct. You know your baby, you know when they aren't right. You won't understand how you know but you'll know. My biggest piece of advice is to join social media groups. The support there is incredible. I wish I had found them sooner. Also contact the reflux charity too. I wish I had done that the first time around. Perhaps I wouldn't have felt quite so alone if I had done both of those with Malachy.

Having a reflux baby is hard. There aren't enough words to describe how hard it is. Please remember that you're not alone. So many of us go through it and we will stand by you while you fight to be heard by health professionals. You're not going crazy, and your baby won't cry forever, but we'll hold your hand while you're in the middle of it, and celebrate when you're through it. You and your baby can do it. I know you can.

16.6   Shauna* & baby

So angry with my GP.

I took my son in this morning after I called the health visitor in tears on Friday because he'd been sick so many times and screamed for pretty much 36 hours. She could hear him over the phone, was lovely and said I needed to get to the doc ASAP.

So I get there and she asks why I've taken an emergency appointment. Umm, because the health visitor told me to... We sit down and I explain what's going on (reflux getting worse) and what they had already given me (ranitidine, Gaviscon). I said we suspect allergies (have been referred to dietician) and said the health visitor had told me to ask what else I could do/give him. I was nearly in tears again, clearly distressed.

She said that "all babies spit up", that he was "doing it for attention" and that I should leave him to cry. She said if I pick him up when he cries, I'm making a rod for my own back and to just get on with it.

In almost the same breath, she said if not eating certain foods helped, I should keep it up. But we had already been through how that was helping with nappies but not reflux.

She was just so unsupportive and unhelpful! I mean, fair enough, she couldn't magically cure him (though we could have tried omeprazole). But as a GP ,she is meant to be on the lookout for PND, if nothing else. Even though I said I was distressed myself, she didn't have anything supportive to say!

I despair of the NHS, I really do.

Oh – and my little man has bloody great bags under his eyes because he keeps waking up crying with reflux pain.

16.7   SARAH & BABY

My baby was diagnosed with silent reflux at 6 weeks and prescribed ranitidine after Gaviscon failed to do anything but cause constipation.

We had been combi feeding from 2 weeks and his symptoms started then. Once diagnosed, we stopped the formula and I managed to get him back to exclusively breastfeeding.

The ranitidine was working great and we had more settled sleep, although he couldn't lie flat or even just have the crib propped up. For weeks on end, he slept in his bouncer chair as it was the only way the acid didn't bother him.

Then the symptoms came back and we tried omeprazole, which just made him worse. Then we were prescribed a combination of lansoprazole and ranitidine at a dosage of ½ a lansoprazole fast tab once a day and 1ml of ranitidine 3 times a day. Then we were referred to a paediatrician.

It was July and baby was 24 weeks before we saw the paediatrician. He said if we'd been referred sooner, he would have suggested early weaning rather than the meds, as he didn't like giving such strong meds to babies. I'd already gotten his ranitidine down to once or twice a day depending on his symptoms, but the doctor said he wanted him off everything by our next appointment in November.

So we started weaning at 26 weeks and gradually I got the ranitidine down to once a day, then started skipping a day, then skipping 2 days, until eventually he was on just the ½ lansoprazole tablet daily. Again, I started skipping days and seeing how he went. I'm proud to say that by 8.5 months, baby was medication-, and more importantly, symptom-free!

We saw the paediatrician last week and were discharged. He was really pleased with us for getting off the meds and very happy in general with how my boy has progressed.

My boy is now 10 months old, eats three meals a day plus snacks, and is still breastfed through the night and on-demand in the day. He is happy and contented, and other than the odd bout of hiccoughs (six times the other day but hadn't had them for weeks before), he is completely symptom-free.

At the beginning, it was so hard – the sleepless nights, screaming baby in pain. I thought it would never end but I want to let you know there is light at the end of the tunnel! Sometimes sooner, sometimes later.

Reflux is awful. It makes you feel hopeless and like a bad parent, because you can't help your baby, but you are doing your best. You are giving all you can to help your little one. You are a brilliant parent! I wish you the happy farewell to reflux that I have had!

AFTERWORD

WHERE TO FROM HERE?

This book has been years in the making. While I have only been writing it for 6 months, the knowledge in it, the research, the questioning of the status quo has been going on for me in some form or another since 2008, with a real kick up the ass when my amazing Sunflower arrived in 2013.

Before I was a parent, I knew parents who had reflux babies. And like most people without a reflux baby, I sort of ignored what they were saying because I could in no way relate.

And then, I had the most unsettled baby in the world, and no-one could relate to me. Without a diagnosis, I did not even know where to look for support or help.

And that was unfair. To my baby. Regardless of karma and what I may or may not have done in any part of my life, here was my perfectly pure and innocent ray of light, in constant agony and pain, and I could do nothing about it.

When I discovered what was going on, and then when Daffodil was born, I was much wiser. Hindsight helped me realise that J and I had a pretty awful experience of the first 12 months of being parents with Sunflower.

And then I started to wonder if my experience was really so exceptional, because I felt we had been treated awfully by those I needed to trust. So in May 2017, I created a survey, with the primary aim of finding out if my experience was way off the norm.

That survey has now had over 1,450 responses and I am sorry to say that my experience seems to be much more "normal" than any healthcare institution would admit.

This survey is propelling me forward. The treatment around reflux babies has got to change. There are better questions and far better solutions to be found much earlier in babies' lives. There is no reason for long-suffering parents to hate being parents. There is no reason for mums to feel they are not listened to. There is no reason for fathers to not know how to support and help their loved ones. There is no reason for families to be pushed to breaking point by the stresses introduced by reflux. There is no reason for this complete lack of support for babies with reflux.

This has got to change. And I plan to change that conversation.

I am not the expert in a lot of this. But I am willing to ask the stupid questions, to challenge the status quo, and to fight for the rights of those babies and families who are too exhausted to do it for themselves; and I will campaign for those who do not yet know reflux may be coming their way.

Parenthood should be an amazing experience. And we all deserve better care and attention to detail from the professionals and systems they employ, even if our babies are on a different development path.

I have a mission to #EradicateBabyReflux as something that destroys families and robs the joy and love from early parenthood. I believe in my heart and soul that by working together, all the families who have lived through it, and all the professionals who work with reflux babies, we can get better answers, quicker for families.

Can you picture a world where, by the age of 6 weeks, most babies' reflux is being managed effectively and appropriately? I can.

And I reckon that the numbers of babies on strong medications will be greatly reduced as a result, making for a stronger and healthier population down the line.

Are you in?

Join me at www.thebabyrefluxlady.co.uk

With love, Áine

ACKNOWLEDGEMENTS

Books are written every day. People manage this all the time. Reflecting on the last 6 months I sometimes wonder how I got it done.

I know how. It has been the support and encouragement of a few very close people who have continuously believed in me, allowed me the space to write, provided me the challenge against my ideas, and encouraged me day in and day out.

The idea of the Baby Reflux Lady's Survival Guide has been in my brain for quite some time, festering there for want of a better term! It has actually been eating me up, knowing what I know, reading the horrific experiences of other reflux families and not being able to help.

I owe the greatest thank you to my amazing husband J, without whom I would not be the person I am today. I would not have seen the person within and I would not have the courage to let her out! His unconditional and unwavering support and strength underpin everything we achieve together; and this book, is indeed, a joint achievement.

My girls, Sunflower and Daffodil, without whom I would never have had reason to learn what I have learned, to be driven to find better answers, and to gather this learning and research into this book. You both challenge me daily, and I love you for it. Because of you both, I am a better person than I ever imagined I could be.

A massive thank you to Kris Emery, my editor. She took my original "book", and crafted my words into a work of pure joy. When I got my book back from her first round of editing, I was incredibly surprised by what I had written – such was the power of Kris's editorial tweaks. She has understood and heard my voice. She has understood my message and made sure that this consistently speaks throughout the book. Thank you, Kris.

Thank you, Nina Ostensen-Hocevar of Ninocka Design. Your illustrations bring a beautiful contrast to the sometimes dark, scary and lonely world of parenthood. I am so grateful to you for understanding the heart of this book and for your friendship. Since we first met, Nina has been one of the people who understood when my sleepless nights continued long past the expected length. I have always adored her artwork, her ability to bring mundane things to life. When I decided to write this book, I knew she would be the person I went to first to bring my thoughts to life.

I want to extend an enormous hug of gratitude to those mums who have shared their stories in this book. Through you, other mums will know they are not alone. The belief in yourselves and your babies, the strength and courage to share your story is amazing. Thank you.

An incredibly big world-sized hug of love and thank you to Suzy Ashworth, my coach. She has stood by my side, pushed me so far past the edge of my comfort zone that I could see the magic on the other side of my internal fears. She has provided constant belief, support, encouragement, challenge and insight, along with a massive amount of practical advice about writing a book and getting it out there. There is no doubt in my mind that without Suzy this book would still be in my head, or at least it would have remained unpublished for a lot longer. Her faith has been steadfast, her actions impeccable and her miracles inspirational.

To my private clients, thank you for letting me into your lives, to help you discover the babies within your babies. You are proof that my approach is applicable and works. Thank you for your trust, your action and your fight for your baby. I know your babies thank you too.

To all those who have supported my work over the last year, blog readers, email readers and internet lurkers, thank you. You let me know there was a need to share my knowledge.

And to the thousands of reflux babies and parents out there, those who I've interacted with over the years, my mission, my manifesto, my calling are because of you. There is a need for the conversation to change. You have shared your more intense, emotional and painful stories with me; you are the reason this book is needed. Thank you for your support.

ABOUT THE AUTHOR

Áine is a mum of two girls, and has first-hand experience of reflux (misdiagnosed and missed) and CMPA in both her daughters. Close to being formally diagnosed with PND, she realised that there was no supportive help coming, no-one was going to listen to her story with care and affection. The love for her daughters was such that she would do anything to protect the health and happiness of her children first, foremost, and forever.

And so, with nothing left to do but take matters into her own hands, Aine did what she knew best – pattern analysis.

A rather unusual combination of Mechanical and Materials Engineering, Maths (not so unusual) and Traditional Chinese Medicine have given Áine a drive to always seek the single cause, the root cause, the one thing that caused this, and this allows her then to identify what is most likely to resolve the issue. This is no different for reflux, colic, CMPA, and other allergies and intolerances in infants.

When everything was dark, there was no more support to ask for and no help coming, Áine had no option but to delve into her reserves and apply the 14-year's experience of professional pattern recognition into an acute awareness of unsettled patterns in young babies.

Áine works tirelessly to change the world for families struggling without support and without answers. She coaches privately, holds individual consultations and can be found blogging and commenting on a growing number of media outlets including Thrive Global and SelfishMother.com. She has been featured in the Mail Online and Mother & Baby Magazine in the UK.

Made in the USA
Coppell, TX
16 April 2024

31390346R00194